"Jessica Yakeley, with unrivalled clinical experience and research insight, distils complex psychoanalytic ideas into a clear, practical guide to antisocial personality disorder. Both accessible and authoritative, this book is indispensable for trainees and experienced clinicians working with antisocial patients".

Peter Fonagy, *Professor of Contemporary Psychoanalysis and Developmental Science, University College London*

"In this compelling book, Yakeley explores the complexities of antisocial personality disorder with unique insight, compassion, and hope. Her rigorous scholarship and clear, concise writing make this book an essential read for everyone interested in understanding this dangerous disorder".

Anna Motz, *Consultant Forensic Psychologist, Author of* A Love that Kills

"Jessica Yakeley, a deeply experienced psychoanalyst and psychiatrist, gives us the most lucid and compelling introduction to the antisocial individual that has ever been penned. Psychoanalysis, like no other theory, helps us understand how their minds work, and there has never been a more important historical moment for such clarity"

J. Reid Meloy, PhD, *Author of* The Psychopathic Mind

Antisocial Personality Disorder

This book offers a vital psychoanalytic overview of antisocial personality disorder, a condition that causes great distress to its sufferers, their families, and society.

Following a historical introduction to how psychoanalysts, from Freud onwards, have conceptualised sociopathy, psychopathy, and delinquency, Jessica Yakeley presents a contemporary psychoanalytic understanding of antisocial personality disorder which integrates current psychoanalytic theory with cutting-edge empirical research findings from developmental and attachment studies. Drawing on her own experience of working with antisocial and violent patients, she offers a psychoanalytic framework to inform clinical work in managing and treating individuals with a diagnosis of this disorder. The reader is introduced to general treatment principles, followed by the latest evidence-based psychoanalytically-informed therapies for the condition. Yakeley also discusses the particular needs and treatment of specific populations of individuals with antisocial personality disorder, including women, sex offenders, and those from ethnic minority backgrounds, addressing issues of race, culture, stigma, and prejudice.

Historically viewed as an untreatable mental disorder, this book offers hope to professionals and patients grappling with antisocial personality disorder, and will be of interest to psychoanalysts, psychiatrists, psychologists, psychotherapists, and other professionals, academics, and trainees working in mental health, criminal justice, and forensic fields.

Jessica Yakeley is a Consultant Psychiatrist in Forensic Psychotherapy and Director of the Portman Clinic, North London Foundation Trust, UK. She is also a training and supervising psychoanalyst of the British Psychoanalytical Society.

Routledge Introductions to Contemporary Psychoanalysis

Series Editor: Aner Govrin
Executive Editor: Yael Peri Herzovich

For more information about this series, please visit: www.routledge.com/Routledge-Introductions-to-Contemporary-Psychoanalysis/book-series/ICP

Antisocial Personality Disorder

A Contemporary Introduction

Jessica Yakeley

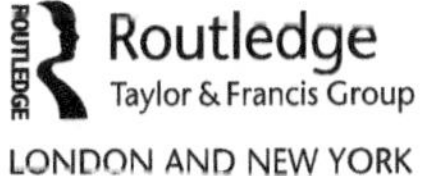

Routledge
Taylor & Francis Group
LONDON AND NEW YORK

Designed cover image: © Michal Heiman, Asylum 1855–2020,
The Sleeper (video, psychoanalytic sofa and Plate 34), exhibition
view, Herzliya Museum of Contemporary Art, 2017

First published 2027
by Routledge
4 Park Square, Milton Park, Abingdon, Oxon OX14 4RN

and by Routledge
605 Third Avenue, New York, NY 10158

*Routledge is an imprint of the Taylor & Francis Group, an informa
business*

© 2027 Jessica Yakeley

For Product Safety Concerns and Information please contact our
EU representative GPSR@taylorandfrancis.com. Taylor & Francis
Verlag GmbH, Kaufingerstraße 24, 80331 München, Germany.

Trademark notice: Product or corporate names may be
trademarks or registered trademarks, and are used only for
identification and explanation without intent to infringe.

British Library Cataloguing-in-Publication Data
A catalogue record for this book is available from the British
Library

ISBN: 978-1-032-90790-1 (hbk)
ISBN: 978-1-032-90158-9 (pbk)
ISBN: 978-1-003-55980-1 (ebk)

DOI: 10.4324/9781003559801

Typeset in Times New Roman
by Taylor & Francis Books

Contents

PART 3
Clinical considerations

PART 4
Special populations

Series Editor's Preface

Aner Govrin

Routledge Introductions to Contemporary Psychoanalysis is one of the most prominent psychoanalytic publishing ventures of our day. The series' aim is to become an encyclopedia of psychoanalysis, with each entry given its own book.

This comprehensive series illuminates the intricate landscape of psychoanalytic theory and practice. In this collection of concise yet illuminating volumes, we delve into the influential figures, groundbreaking concepts, and transformative theories that shape the contemporary psychoanalytic landscape.

At the heart of each volume lies a commitment to clarity, accessibility, and depth. Our expert authors, renowned scholars and practitioners in their respective fields, guide readers through the complexities of psychoanalytic thought with precision and enthusiasm. Whether you are a seasoned psychoanalyst, a student eager to explore the field, or a curious reader seeking insight into the human psyche, our series offers a wealth of knowledge and insight.

Each volume serves as a gateway into a specific aspect of psychoanalytic theory and practice. From the pioneering works of Sigmund Freud to the innovative contributions of modern theorists such as Antonino Ferro and Michal Eigen, our series covers a diverse range of topics, including seminal figures, key concepts, and emerging trends. Whether you are interested in classical psychoanalysis, object relations theory, or the intersection of neuroscience and psychoanalysis, you will find a wealth of resources within our collection.

One of the hallmarks of our series is its interdisciplinary approach. While rooted in psychoanalytic theory, our volumes draw upon insights from psychology, philosophy, sociology, and other disciplines to offer a holistic understanding of the human mind and its complexities.

Each volume in the series is crafted with the reader in mind, balancing scholarly rigor with engaging prose. Whether you are embarking on your journey into psychoanalysis or seeking to deepen your understanding of specific topics, our series provides a clear and comprehensive roadmap.

Moreover, our series is committed to fostering dialogue and debate within the psychoanalytic community. Each volume invites readers to critically engage with the material, encouraging reflection, discussion, and further exploration.

We invite you to join us on this journey of discovery as we explore the ever-evolving landscape of psychoanalysis.

Aner Govrin

Acknowledgements

This book would not have been possible without my colleagues, past and present, at the Portman Clinic, who have taught me so much about working with antisocial and violent patients. Particular thanks to Stephen Blumenthal, my co-therapist and partner in crime, for the group we run for men with antisocial personality disorder; to Gabrielle Brown, for keeping me sane; and to Stan Ruszczynski, my predecessor as Director, who took a risk 15 years ago in letting me start the group in the first place.

I'm also grateful to Peter Fonagy and Anthony Bateman, who went with my idea of doing a trial of mentalisation-based treatment for this population thought of as untreatable, which we proved to be erroneous despite expectations to the contrary. Thanks also to my friends and colleagues in the wider world of forensic psychotherapy, in particular Anne Aiyegbusi, Gwen Adshead, Anna Motz, and Estela Welldon; and to Reid Meloy for teaching me everything I know about psychopathy.

However, the most important teachers have been the patients themselves, who have bravely and movingly engaged in therapy, allowed me into the subjectivity and suffering of their lives, and opened themselves up to the possibility of change.

Finally, thanks to Bryn, who gave me the support and space to write this book and provided an essential external perspective.

Introduction

The psychopath is a familiar and enduring figure in literature, film, and journalism, whether as the cold-blooded serial killer, mafia gangster, ruthless tycoon, or Nazi SS officer. Their superficial charm, ruthlessness, pathological lying, emotional detachment, lack of remorse, and capacity for sadistic violence excites and fascinates the public imagination, popularising and glamourising the lives, adventures, and exploits of such individuals.

However, people living with a diagnosis of antisocial personality disorder (ASPD), which includes the construct of psychopathy, may experience considerable distress, as well as cause significant harm to others. ASPD is a relatively common condition, its prevalence ranging from around 1% to 6.8% in the general population, and it is significantly elevated in criminal justice settings, where up to 80% of prisoners may meet diagnostic criteria. It is strongly associated with violent behaviour and is a robust predictor of future violence, reconviction, reincarceration, and recidivism. ASPD is associated with considerable morbidity, commonly co-occurring with anxiety and depression, as well as substance misuse, and is linked to poor physical health and increased early mortality due to suicide, drug misuse, and reckless behaviour. Individuals with the condition also exert a heavy toll on others, with negative impacts on their families and relationships with others, as well as increased involvement with social services and the health and criminal justice systems. The associated financial burden to society, including victim injury, property damage, lost employment, and service costs, is considerable.

DOI: 10.4324/9781003559801-1

ASPD is a complex multifactorial mental disorder which may be understood from a variety of perspectives. This book offers a psychoanalytic approach, but this is just one framework for understanding and treating the condition, and it aims to complement, rather than replace, other psychological, social, and biological models and fields of research. Clinical vignettes of disguised or fictionalised patients are provided to illustrate the text.

The first two chapters trace the historical evolution of theory within the psychoanalytic literature on the origins, development, and clinical manifestations of antisocial, criminal, and psychopathic behaviour. Chapter 1 explores Freud's notion of "criminals from a sense of guilt" – individuals who are drawn to committing forbidden antisocial deeds to relieve a pre-existing unconscious sense of Oedipal guilt. This inspired the theories of subsequent early psychoanalytic pioneers, including Fenichel, Greenacre, Horney, Reich, and Klein about people who displayed antisocial and psychopathic character traits and behaviour, highlighting failures of the superego, deficits in early identifications, and early disturbed parent-child relations. However, with the exception of Melanie Klein, these psychoanalytic writers inferred their ideas regarding the roots of antisociality and psychopathy from the analysis of adult patients.

Chapter 2 reviews the parallel development during the first half of the 20th century of research into juvenile delinquency based on direct observations of children in the context of the child guidance movement, which was heavily influenced by psychoanalytic ideas. Instead of viewing psychopathy and antisocial behaviour as being primarily due to constitutional deficits, prominent psychoanalysts such as Anna Freud, with her concept of social maladjustment; Winnicott, in his descriptions of the privation, deprivation, and the antisocial tendency; and Bowlby, with his "affectionless psychopaths", highlighted disturbances in the mother-infant relationship and viewed antisociality and psychopathy as defences against early trauma.

The following three chapters document the progression and integration of these earlier psychoanalytic theories into current conceptualisations of ASPD. Chapter 3 presents the confusion surrounding the diagnosis of ASPD in relation to psychopathy and reviews the current state of research outside of the psycho-analytic field on the role of neurobiological, genetic, and environ-mental factors into the aetiology of these conditions within the framework of attachment theory. Chapter 4 introduces a con-temporary understanding of psychopathy, which integrates psycho-analytic object relations theory with attachment and biological research and demonstrates how the psychopathic personality emer-ges via failures of internalisation and identification, disturbed inter-nal object relations, and the development of a psychopathic superego. Chapter 5 focusses on the broader diagnostic category of ASPD, through the lens of mentalisation, one of the most influential frameworks for understanding normal and pathological human relationships to emerge from psychoanalysis and attachment theory in recent years. This chapter considers how ASPD can be considered as a disorder of attachment and mentalisation, and how specific deficits in the mentalising capacities of individuals with ASPD mean they display a lack of empathy, emotional instability, and are more prone to impulsive, aggressive, and violent behaviour.

The next two chapters address clinical work with patients who have a diagnosis of ASPD, illustrated with anonymised clinical vignettes. Chapter 6 applies a psychoanalytic framework to for-mulate general principles of the assessment and treatment of ASPD. This includes risk assessment, the influence of counter-transference in the setting in which treatment occurs, evaluation of psychopathy and other personality traits which predict treatment response, and how to engage the patient in a therapeutic process. Chapter 7 reviews the evidence for the treatment of ASPD, and specific psychoanalytically-informed therapies that have been adapted for patients with the disorder, focussing on individual psychodynamic psychotherapy, group analytic therapy, and mentalisation-based treatment (MBT).

The last three chapters look at particular populations under the ASPD diagnostic umbrella. Chapter 8 offers a psychoanalytic understanding of antisocial, violent, and psychopathic women and how they differ from their male counterparts in their tendencies to dissociate and deceive, and how they are more likely to direct their aggression towards their children or partners, who are used as vehicles for the expression of unconscious conflict, stemming from early experiences of parental neglect and abuse. Chapter 9 proposes that psychoanalytic ideas on perversion and sexual deviance may provide insights into the psychosexual behaviour of the sex offender with ASPD, the central premise being that harmful sexual acts towards others may be conceptualised as defences against unconscious anxieties and aggression.

The final chapter addresses ASPD and race. People of colour are overrepresented in the criminal justice system, and those with ASPD may be doubly disadvantaged, not only by stigma and prejudice but by the racism that exists at both individual and systemic levels. This chapter explores contemporary psychoanalytic theories of racism and how these might be applied to working with antisocial patients. Concepts such as whiteness, racist psychic organisations, internal racism, and black rage are discussed in relation to understanding conscious and unconscious racist attitudes and behaviours of professionals and institutions, as well as how issues of racism manifest in therapy, including racist transference and countertransference phenomena.

In writing this book, I have drawn on my own clinical work as a psychiatrist and forensic psychotherapist with patients with the diagnosis of ASPD at the Portman Clinic, where I also teach and supervise other professionals who manage and treat antisocial offenders within the criminal justice system, and my involvement in a randomised controlled trial of mentalisation-based treatment for offenders with ASPD in the UK National Probation Service. The book challenges the long-standing and persistent belief that people with ASPD are untreatable and aims to provide understanding, insight, and hope to those individuals, their families, and the professionals involved in their care.

Part 1

Historical overview

Chapter 1

Antisocial personalities

Historical perspectives

Moral degeneration

Prior to the 19th century, criminals were seen as sinners deserving punishment, deportation, or execution (Simonsen, 2022). In 1801, the French psychiatrist Philippe Pinel first described individuals with impulsive, destructive behaviours but no intellectual defects as "manie sans délire" (Pinel, 1806). The American psychiatrist Benjamin Rush similarly noted these traits but rejected the idea they were immoral (Rush, 1812). In 1835, the British psychiatrist Robert Cowell Prichard, supported by the British psychiatrist Henry Maudsley, introduced the concept of "moral insanity" to describe individuals with severe moral and emotional disturbances but without any deficiency in intellect or psychotic symptoms (Prichard, 1835). Augustine Morel, a French psychiatrist, expanded these ideas by introducing hereditary explanations of the disorder (Morel, 1857), laying the foundation for the Italian psychiatrist Cesare Lombroso's concept of the *delinquente nato* or "born criminal". Lombroso attributed the behaviour of some murderers to neurobiological abnormalities, claiming such factors explained around 25% of cases (Lombroso, 1911). These evolving theories shaped early psychiatric and legal views on criminality.

The idea of a biologically rooted entity that was degenerative in moral stature continued to gain traction in the later 19th century, when the term "psychopathic" first appeared in psychiatric nomenclature. In 1891, Julius Koch, a German philosopher and psychiatrist, introduced the term "constitutional psychopathic

DOI: 10.4324/9781003559801-3

inferiority" to describe such individuals, which was based on the concept of psychopathy, meaning "sick mind". Psychopathy, however, was an ill-defined term, prompting subsequent German psychiatrists, most notably Emil Kraeplin, a prominent descriptive psychopathologist (Simonsen, 2022), to differentiate discrete types. Psychopathic personality became an overarching term for all disorders of personality, within which he defined four different categories of criminal according to psychological and sociological criteria: morbid liars and swindlers, criminals by impulse, professional criminals, and morbid vagabonds.

In 1923, Kurt Schneider, another influential German psychiatrist, further classified psychopathic personalities based on their phenomenology but in contrast to his predecessors stressed a value-free system whereby different personality types were based on psychological principles that were independent of societal ideas of morality. He was also the first to use a trait-based model of character pathology, proposing that abnormal personalities were extreme variants of normal personalities.

Thus, the beginning of the 20th century heralded a psychological interest divorced from moral judgement in antisocial personalities and behaviours. This paved the way for the new discipline of psychoanalysis to extend its reach to matters of criminology and the law. Freud's revolutionary ideas now focussed attention away from the moral standards of society towards the individual's internal conflicts, which, he proposed, were intimately linked to the forbidden fantasies of infantile sexuality.

Freud: Criminals from a sense of guilt

Freud's understanding of criminality was centred on the idea that antisocial acts represent the externalisation of an unconscious sense of guilt, which is linked to the superego and the Oedipus complex. Although his best-known paper on the subject is *Criminals from a Sense of Guilt* (Freud, 1916), his interest in the psychopathology of antisocial behaviour and criminality is evident in his earlier and later works.

In 1906, at the invitation of Professor Löffler, a professor of jurisprudence in Vienna, Freud gave a lecture titled *Psycho-analysis and the Establishment of the Facts in Legal Proceedings* (Freud, 1906) in which he drew an analogy between the criminal and the hysteric. In both individuals, he said, there is a secret. However, in the criminal it is a secret that he is consciously aware of and which he hides from others; but in the hysteric, the secret is hidden not only from others but also from himself. The hysteric's secret consists of ideas and memories strongly associated with affect but which are deemed unacceptable to his conscious mind and are thus pushed out of consciousness. This repressed psychical material, which Freud thought was invariably of a sexual nature, generates somatic and psychical symptoms that plague the hysteric like a guilty conscience. The hysteric is genuinely ignorant of the secret origin of his symptoms, whereas in the case of criminal, his ignorance is pretence.

Freud elaborated on the nature of unconscious guilt in *Some Character-Types Met with in Psycho-analytic Work*, the third essay of *Criminals from a Sense of Guilt* (Freud, 1916). He describes a group of individuals who are drawn to committing forbidden antisocial deeds to relieve a pre-existing unconscious sense of guilt. In such criminals, as in naughty children, the guilt does not arise from the crime; on the contrary, the crime committed arises from the guilt and thus serves to provoke punishment to assuage the guilt and relieve the criminal's suffering. Freud proposed that this unconscious guilt is intimately connected with the Oedipus complex and is a reaction to "the two great criminal intentions of killing the father and having sexual relations with the mother" (Freud, 1916, p. 332), which he believed are the two original crimes at the basis of humanity (Freud, 1913).

The superego now becomes a central psychic structure in the psychopathology of the criminal. The superego is a mental agency or structure which Freud introduced in his structural model of the mind (Freud, 1923). The superego develops from the id and ego during childhood and contains the person's ideals, conscience, and moral values. It is formed via an early narcissistic identification and internalisation of parental moral values and prohibitions around the age of 4 or 5 as a resolution of the Oedipus conflict. It is a more rigid structure than the id or ego and acts like an internal judge presiding over the ego, presenting ideals to it, observing and criticising it. Consciousness of guilt is an expression of conflict between the ego and superego.

With Freud's introduction of the death instinct in his final theory of the instincts (Freud, 1920), he developed the idea of unconscious guilt in his theories of masochism and sadism. Some individuals develop a harsh and inflexible superego. Here, the person unconsciously adopts a punitive and judgemental attitude to himself, resulting in an unconscious masochistic tendency to suffer. Freud discovered that the formation of such a severe superego is not solely dependent upon experiencing and internalising harsh parental attitudes in early childhood but could arise in individuals who had experienced more benign parenting. Freud proposed that the presence of a very harsh superego is due to an excess of the death instinct that is channelled through the superego (Freud, 1930).

Freud (1924) described another form of masochism, moral masochism, as a form of unconscious suffering driven by guilt rather than erotic pleasure. These individuals act against their own interests, often to provoke punishment, without awareness of their pleasure in suffering. The sadistic superego is conscious, while the ego's masochism remains unconscious. This dynamic reflects a regressive return to the Oedipus complex and repressed incestuous desire. Some criminals may be moral masochists, offending repeatedly to sustain this unconscious need for chastisement.

When the death instinct dominates, superego development is impaired, reducing internal conflict. Aggression is directed outward, forming the basis of sadism, unlike the inward focus of moral masochism. In *Dostoyevsky and Parricide* (1928), his study of the Russian writer's great work, Freud identified three criminal types: primal criminal, whose crime assuages their unconscious sense of guilt; the political or religious criminal, and the common criminal.

The common criminal does not seek castigation for his offence but "commits crimes without any sense of guilt, who have either developed no moral inhibitions or who, in their conflict with society, consider themselves justified in their action" (Freud, 1916, p. 333). In *Dostoyevsky and Parricide*, Freud wrote further, "two traits are essential in a criminal: boundless egoism and a strong destructive urge. Common to both of these, and a necessary condition for their expression, is absence of love, lack of an emotional appreciation of (human) objects" (Freud, 1928. p. 178). And two years later, in a footnote in *Civilisation and its Discontents* (Freud, 1930), Freud drew on Aichhorn's study of delinquency, *Wayward Youth* (Aichhorn, 1965 [1925]), to contrast the two main types of pathological parenting: the overly indulgent father who contributes to the formation of an excessively harsh superego by suppressing external expression of aggression; and the unloved delinquent child who lacks this inner conflict and directs aggression outward.

In both these texts, Freud highlighted how it is not just the constitutional strength of the instincts which determines whether a person becomes criminal or delinquent, but this also depends on the role of the environment, and whether the child receives parental love. Where such love is lacking, aggression is directed outwards, the superego remains underdeveloped, and the person is unable to form emotionally meaningful relationships with others. Freud's ideas here herald two key themes that are further developed in the early psychoanalytic literature on the genesis of the antisocial character – the nature of superego development and the role of the maternal object.

The early Freudians

The interwar period was fertile for the psychoanalytic study of the criminal. Criminology was emerging as a distinct discipline, and psychoanalytic thinking exerted a significant influence on its development in the early 20th century. Freud's theories attracted the interest of his early adherents in Vienna, such as Paul Federn, in his studies on the psychology of sadism and masochism (Federn, 1913; 1919); Theodor Reik, in his study of the psychology of murder and how criminals tended to betray themselves by means of slips of the tongue (Reik, 1925; 1932); Fenichel, with his delineation of the "instinct-ridden" character, who commits crimes at the mercy of a projected superego and sense of guilt (Fenichel, 1945); and Alfred Adler, who, in contrast to Freud's emphasis on unconscious motivations and Oedipal conflict, proposed that social influences, particularly the dynamics of power and compensation, shape the personality of the neurotic criminal, whose illegal acts are an attempt to overcompensate for an inferiority complex caused by parental neglect (Adler, 1924).

Such ideas began to influence psychoanalysts and criminologists in other European cities beyond Vienna. In Budapest, Sandor Ferenczi, in his early work as a forensic medical expert, introduced psychoanalytic concepts to the legal profession, cautioning that the criminal's motivations for his offence lay in his unconscious, not in his conscious confessions (Ferenczi, 1919). In Berlin, Franz Alexander similarly argued for psychoanalytic thinking, and the notion of the unconscious, in the courtroom. His interest in criminology stemmed from his analysis of a woman with kleptomania, following Freud's cases described in *Some Character-Types Met with in Psychoanalytic Work* (Freud, 1916). He designated some criminals as having what he termed a "neurotic character" in which the neurotic element in such individuals is evident not so much in the form of symptoms but pervades their personality, thus influencing their behaviour (Alexander, 1930). Alexander began working with Hugo Staub, a prominent criminologist, and their textbook *The Criminal, the Judge and the Public: A Psychological Analysis* (Alexander & Staub, 1931) attracted the interest of judges and criminal lawyers throughout Germany. They argued that such criminals should not be held legally responsible for their crimes, as they are the result of unconscious forces rather than rational thought and recommended psychoanalytic treatment in opposition to punishment, which would unconsciously gratify more masochistic offenders.

Klein: The harsh and sadistic superego

Following Freud, these early psychoanalysts emphasised the pathological Oedipal dynamics and deficits in superego formation present in criminals. However, others dissented from Freud, proposing that rather than the superego being rudimentary or absent altogether in such individuals, it is present and its strength, not its weakness, results in criminal tendencies. Otto Fenichel believed there was some evidence of primitive superego formation in psychopaths, whose faulty character development results from a strong pregenital fixation of the Oedipus complex (Fenichel, 1931). But it was Melanie Klein who significantly departed from Freud; in her view, far from criminal behaviour being due to an absent superego, its excessive harshness and severity forms the origin of antisociality and deviance.

Unlike Freud, Melanie Klein believed the Oedipus complex began much earlier, around the end of the first year of life. Before this stage, the infant experiences terrifying phantasies of a combined parental figure, imagining the mother's body as containing the father's penis and rival babies engaged in constant, sadistic intercourse. These phantasies occur within the "paranoid-schizoid position", where the infant, overwhelmed by life and death instincts, projects love and hate onto split versions of the self and mother: idealised "good" and persecutory "bad" objects. These are introjected and reprojected in a cycle that gradually leads to the "depressive position". In this more integrated state, the infant begins to experience ambivalence, guilt, loss, and the capacity for mourning and gratitude. This shift allows the child to enter the Oedipus complex more fully, with the eventual relinquishing of Oedipal desires as part of emotional maturation.

Departing from Freud's structural theory in which the superego is formed due to the resolution of the Oedipus complex, Klein asserted that primitive superego figures develop from the beginning of life in response to the child's infantile sadistic phantasies of attacking the parental couple and killing the rival parent, which are projected into external objects and then experienced by the child as persecutory and forbidding, dynamics that are integral to the paranoid-schizoid position. In her papers *Criminal Behaviour in Normal Children* (Klein, 1927) and *On Criminality* (Klein, 1934), Klein proposed that criminal tendencies are present in all children as the manifestation of these sadistic phantasies, resulting in a harsh early superego, which gradually becomes less severe in normal development as the child matures and experiences guilt for their sadistic attacks. However, in some individuals, due to innate constitutional factors and the dominance of the death drive, the early severe superego does not become modified but becomes abnormally destructive, engendering paranoid-schizoid persecutory anxieties and guilt, which are unconsciously projected outwards in the form of aggression or criminal acts which consequently need to be punished. In contrast to Freud, therefore, it is the presence of a very harsh superego, rather than an absent superego, which can drive someone to commit crime.

Psychopathy: Entitlement, exploitation, and deception

As psychoanalysis expanded its interest from the genesis of discrete neurotic illnesses to character pathology, several other early psychoanalysts made significant contributions to the delineation of a psychopathic personality type, focussing on phenomenology and psychodynamics. These were influenced by the American psychiatrist Hervey Milton Cleckley's seminal book *The Mask of Sanity* (Cleckley, 1941). Cleckley described 16 behavioural and psychological criteria for psychopathy, including guiltlessness, lack of remorse and shame, incapacity for object love, emotional shallowness, impulsivity, egocentricity, inability to learn from experience, and lack of insight. He believed that people with psychopathy could appear normal, but this was a mask which concealed an underlying psychosis. He differentiated psychopathy as a mental disorder distinct from criminality and asserted that the psychopathic personalities are not all criminals but are also prevalent in successful and respected professionals including businessmen, scientists, and doctors. The primary traits of the psychopath identified by Cleckley were later empirically defined and measured by the psychologist Robert Hare (1991) in the development of his widely-used risk assessment tool, the Psychopathy Check List.

The psychoanalysts Otto Fenichel (1945), Wilhelm Reich (1945), and Karen Horney (1945), in their books on character pathology published in the same year, provided rich descriptions of the attitudes and behaviours of certain character types that are akin to Cleckley's description of psychopathy.

Fenichel (1945) elaborated on his concept of the "instinct ridden character" in which there are deficits and distortions of early identifications, and instinctual strivings escape the inhibiting influences of the superego. These individuals manage their self-esteem with denial and a veneer of perfection, to defend against narcissistic injury. Reich identified a "phallic-narcissistic character" type, a psychopathic personality who is arrested in the phallic phase of psychosexual development and exhibits aggressive and sadistic behaviour, especially towards women, which provides direct gratification in the absence of reaction formation but also serves as a narcissistic defence against regression to the passive and anal stages (Reich, 1945).

The neo-Freudian psychoanalyst Karen Horney accepted many of Freud's basic concepts but gave more emphasis to childhood relational experiences, rather than instinctual vicissitudes, in determining the formation of personality. In her theory of neurotic personalities, she identified the "sadistic personality", whose defining features include exploiting, triumphing over, thwarting, disparaging, and humiliating others, behaviour which she attributed to an externalisation of the person's self-loathing, senses of futility and alienation from life, and failure to live up to idealised standards. She also emphasised the presence of anxiety, not solely arising from a lack of a sense of safety due to adverse environmental factors in childhood but also due to a fear of the destructive aspects of himself and of retaliation from others.

Phyllis Greenacre, an American psychoanalyst, published two seminal papers on psychopathy. In *Conscience in the Psychopath* (1945), she supported Klein's view on early aggression and anxiety shaping the superego but argued this only led to psychopathy when combined with later relational factors. She observed that psychopathic patients often have narcissistic parents – stern, distant fathers and indulgent, superficial mothers. The child is valued for appearances, not individuality, which delays separation and individuation. Love is inhibited, and unconscious aggression emerges. During the Oedipal phase, maternal overinvolvement and paternal austerity hinder paternal identification, fostering ambivalence towards authority. This dynamic underlies the psychopath's superficial charm and impaired reality testing.

In a later paper, *The Imposter*, Greenacre elaborated on the consequences of the psychopath's failure in Oedipal identifications, identification with an aggressive and narcissistic parent, and defences against maternal annihilation, which result in the conscious imitation and unconscious simulation of other's thoughts, emotions, and behaviours, as well as a strong sense of voyeurism and exhibitionism, sexual relations distorted by sadomasochistic excitement, and a compulsion to commit fraud (Greenacre, 1958).

Greenacre's paper on the imposter drew on the work of the Polish American psychoanalyst and member of Freud's inner circle, Helene Deutsch. Deutsch described the "as-if" personality, a schizoid type character who relates to others based on "pseudo contacts" and "ungenuine pseudo emotions" as a substitute for a real feeling of connection (Deutsch, 1934). In a later paper, titled *The Imposter: Contribution to Ego Psychology of a Type of Psychopath* (Deutsch, 1955), she described the analysis of a psychopathic patient whose inflated ego ideals, passive entitlement, and grandiose fantasies, stemming from his experience of a successful and dominant father and an indulgent and anxious mother, led to a pretence that he was successful, a stance that broke down during treatment when his underlying anxiety and feelings of inferiority were unmasked.

Personality organisations

Melanie Klein (1975 [1957]; 1964), Edith Jacobson (1964; 1971), and Margaret Mahler (1968; 1979) also made important contributions to understanding psychopathy from an object-relational perspective. However, the American psychiatrist and psychoanalyst Kernberg (1976; 1984) has arguably had the greatest influence in the fields of psychiatry and personality disorder, advancing the idea that psychopathy represents a severe form of narcissistic personality disorder. Kernberg's concept of personality organisation is valuable for understanding the development of traits that predispose an individual to psychopathy. He adopts a dimensional approach, suggesting that there are three levels of personality organisation, ranging from relatively healthy to severely impaired: neurotic, borderline, and psychotic levels. These levels are distinguished based on identity integration, the nature of the individual's defence mechanisms, and their ability to test reality.

The neurotic level represents the most mature and healthiest form of personality organisation. Individuals at this level have intact reality testing and the ability to gain insight, with a consistent and integrated sense of themselves and others. They typically rely on mature defence mechanisms, such as repression, when under stress. On the opposite end of the personality organisation spectrum is the psychotic level, which refers to individuals with severely disorganised personalities who struggle to distinguish the boundaries between themselves and others, as well as between internal experiences and perceptions versus those originating in the external world. These individuals primarily rely on immature defences, such as denial, projection, and splitting – defences that are normal in young children but become pathological when they dominate adult behaviour.

Between the neurotic and psychotic levels lies the borderline level of personality organisation. Unlike individuals at the more severe psychotic level, those at the borderline level generally have intact reality testing. However, they experience a fragmented sense of self and others, with a diffuse and incoherent identity, which leads to relationships that are often superficial, narcissistically driven, and lacking in empathy. These individuals fail to recognise others as distinct individuals with different needs and viewpoints. They predominantly rely on primitive defence mechanisms such as splitting, projective identification, idealisation, denigration, and omnipotent control. Kernberg suggests that the psychopath's character is organised at the more severe end of the borderline level. While the psychopath may appear to function at a more sophisticated level – Cleckley's "mask of sanity" – this conceals deeper and pervasive deficits in their psychological structure and functioning.

From drives to object relations

In this chapter, we have seen how Freud's original notion that the externalisation of unconscious Oedipal guilt drives criminal behaviour was elaborated on by his early adherents, who emphasised the failure of identifications and the centrality of the superego in the development of a psychopathic character. We can also observe a theoretical shift from Freud's drive model of the mind, where criminality is determined by the constitutional strength of the life and death instincts towards an object relations model in which the importance of the child's early relationships and the role of environmental factors become more evident in the development of a criminal or psychopathic personality. However, except for Klein, most of the forementioned psychoanalysts derived their theories from the treatment of adults, inferring the causative factors of antisocial characters from their patients' histories rather than from therapeutic work with children. The next chapter will explore the psychoanalytic study of juvenile delinquency and the contributions of psychoanalysts whose theories of antisocial behaviour arose from their direct observation and treatment of troubled children and adolescents who had been separated or traumatised by their early caregivers, experiences which in some constituted the precursors to criminality in adulthood.

Chapter 2

Juvenile delinquency

The child guidance movement

The advent of the 20th century signalled a growing interest in psychological and social approaches to juvenile delinquency and the evolution of the child guidance movement, which was influenced by psychoanalytic ideas from its inception. This movement was initiated by the British American psychiatrist and criminologist William Healy in Chicago in 1906 to end the imprisonment of children and develop multidisciplinary clinics to treat children and youths with behavioural and mental disorders. Healy was an early proponent of psychoanalysis in the United States and developed a research programme studying 4000 juvenile delinquents in the juvenile court system (Healy, 1915). In his interviews with these young people, he was struck by how many had experienced what he referred to as "defective home conditions".

The child guidance movement spread outside of the United States, first to Vienna, where Alfred Adler started the first child guidance clinic in 1919. This gained the attention of August Aichhorn, an Austrian educator who was encouraged by Anna Freud to train as a psychoanalyst and subsequently established a child guidance service for the Vienna Psychoanalytic Society in 1922. Like Healy, Aichhorn viewed delinquency as stemming not just from inherited traits but also from early parental relationships and societal failures. He saw delinquency as a developmental arrest, where the ego remains dominated by the pleasure principle. This could result from either parental overindulgence or harshness, both of

DOI: 10.4324/9781003559801-4

which hinder ego and superego development, predisposing children to act out more frequently than those whose egos are governed by the reality principle. Dysfunctional homes further reinforce delinquency, where the parents' aggressive behaviour becomes incorporated into the child's ego ideal.

Aichhorn made a crucial distinction between what he called "manifest delinquency" – that is, the overt and observable anti-social behaviours – and "latent delinquency" – the underlying unconscious conflicts which need to be addressed. He warned that punishment solely suppresses the delinquent behaviours, which can only improve if the unconscious dynamics are understood. Aichhorn developed his own distinctive, intuitive, and idiosyncratic treatment of aggressive and antisocial youths, involving modifications of psychoanalytic technique, including manipulations of the transference; for example, mobilising or diminishing guilt feelings in the child by asking him for symbolic favours such as buying Aichhorn a newspaper or packet of cigarettes.

The ISTD and the Portman Clinic

The first child guidance clinic was established in the UK in 1927 by the child psychiatrist Emanuel Miller, who, with other key figures within psychiatry, psychoanalysis, and criminology, was instrumental in setting up the Institute for the Scientific Treatment of Delinquency (ISTD). The aims of the ISTD were to develop and promote scientific research into the causes and prevention of crime, as well as establish observation centres and clinics for the diagnosis and treatment of delinquency and crime. The ISTD marked the union of two strands within the new discipline of criminology – the humanitarian, which promoted treating rather than punishing offenders; and the scientific, in the empirical investigation of the different theories and treatments of delinquency prevalent at the time (Saville & Rumney, 1992). The ISTD was founded in 1931 by Grace Pailthorpe, a psychoanalyst and psychiatrist, and later surrealist painter, who had conducted research into the psychology of female offenders incarcerated in prison and religious institutions for young women for offences of delinquency, theft, promiscuity, and prostitution. Pailthorpe enlisted the interest of psychoanalysts such as Edward Glover and Kate Friedlander, as well as the support of other prominent figures, including Havelock Ellis, Sigmund Freud, Carl Jung, Otto Rank, Bronislaw Malinowski, H.G. Wells, the Chief Rabbi, the Archbishop of York, and the Dean of Canterbury. The ISTD and its clinical arm, the Psychopathic Clinic, which later became the Portman Clinic, now formed the centre for psychoanalytic research into the causes and treatment of juvenile delinquency, as well as violent and antisocial behaviour in adults, in the second quarter of the 20th century.

The Portman Clinic's direct clinical work with children and adolescents played a part in shifting aetiological theories towards recognising the role of the child's environment in the development of delinquency and criminality, rather than innate biological factors, as advanced by Freud and Klein. One of the most vociferous of Klein's opponents was her own daughter, Melitta Schmideberg, who was an active member of the ISTD and Portman Clinic and made a significant contribution to the psychoanalytic literature on criminality and delinquency, as well as child psychoanalysis. Initially collaborating with her mother professionally, by the early 1930s she started to show more independent ideas, particularly regarding the intersection between the patient's internal world and their relation to the external world, and how difficulties in the child could represent failures in the mother rather than being due to the persecutory phantasies of the child. Working with delinquent children, she contended that anxiety, rather than aggression, underlay delinquent acts, and that projection failed in its role of relieving anxiety and as a driving force for development if the external environment itself was unfavourable, in terms of the negative attitudes and behaviours of parental figures (Schmideberg, 1935).

Kate Friedlander, another psychoanalyst at the Portman Clinic, made key contributions to understanding delinquency. After working in a Berlin juvenile court, she fled to London in 1933, collaborated with Anna Freud at the Hampstead Clinic, and later founded a child guidance clinic in West Sussex. Influenced by Aichhorn, she viewed delinquency as a failure of social adaptation, proposing that some children possess a latent personality structure marked by a weak ego, unmodified instinctual drives, and a dependent superego. While not inherently delinquent, these traits, combined with adverse environments, could lead to delinquency. She emphasised the mother-child relationship as the central environmental influence, suggesting that factors like poverty, housing, and unemployment affect delinquency primarily through their impact on this relationship.

Maternal separation and deprivation

The effects of ruptures in the child's relationship with his earliest caregivers in the development of psychopathic character traits became an area of empirical study for psychoanalytic researchers in the United States during the interwar period. The American psychiatrist and psychoanalyst David Levy studied adopted children who had suffered maternal rejection. He coined the term "affect hunger" to describe the emotional hunger for maternal love, care, and protection that results from a lack of maternal affection. This can lead to a chronic emotional detachment and incapacity to bond, sometimes concealed behind a façade of normality – a deficiency disease of the emotional life akin to bodily illness caused by a lack of vital nutritional elements (Levy, 1937).

Lauretta Bender, an early American pioneer of child psychiatry, drew on Anna Freud's and others' work to understand the psychopathology of institutionalised children (Bender, 1947). She observed children who had spent prolonged periods in institutions where there were no opportunities to develop affectional ties with adults or had been passed from one foster home to the next. These children showed an inability to form relationships or identify with others, with disturbances in intellectual, emotional, and social aspects of the personality, including antisocial behaviour. She postulated that the children's developmental processes became fixated at the earliest stage, the ego was defective, there was no superego, and internal impulses were unmodified and demanded immediate satisfaction. The younger the child at the age of deprivation, the more serious the psychopathology. Such children did not respond to punishment, discipline, or therapy because they could not form a therapeutic relationship.

However, it was the Second World War which brought new insights into the deleterious consequences on children of being separated from their parents due to evacuation, and how those who had already experienced parental discord or deprivation were more likely to exhibit aggressive or delinquent behaviour. Observation of these children influenced the work of Anna Freud, Donald Winnicott, and John Bowlby, which built on the growing awareness of the centrality of maternal love for healthy child development and effected a shift in psychoanalytic theory from an intrapsychic model towards an object-relational paradigm.

Anna Freud: Social maladjustment

Anna Freud made significant contributions to the field of child psychoanalysis. Whilst remaining loyal to her father's overall metapsychology, she elaborated on his theories through her direct observation of school and nursery children, including those with delinquency. She was one of the pioneers of using naturalistic observations of children to research child development as opposed to basing theory on the reconstructed child from the analyses of adults. In 1941, with Dorothy Burlingham, she established the Hampstead War Nursery for children whose lives had been disrupted by the war and observed firsthand the effects of loss and separation on children and their families. Her work on the theory and technique of child psychoanalysis was developed over 50 years and included her ideas on "socially maladjusted" children, including psychopathic children.

Drawing on both her father's instinct theory and subsequent object relations theory, Anna Freud viewed delinquent behaviour in children as a manifestation of failures of the phases in normal social development, which progress from attachment to the parents through relationships with teachers and other children at nursery and school, and finally to adaptation to the cultural standards of the community. Following Aichhorn's findings in the histories of the antisocial and delinquent children he treated, she believed that in most of such cases there has been an absent, neglectful, or emotionally unstable mother, or the early care of the infant was provided by impersonal or changing figures. The transformation of narcissistic libido to object libido is subsequently impeded, leading to withdrawal to bodily auto-erotic pleasures, under-development of the ego and superego due to deficient identifications, and inadequate binding of the child's aggressive impulses. These impulses then manifest in destructive or antisocial behaviour rather than being channelled, neutralised, and sublimated with the development of higher-level defences during the Oedipal period.

Anna Freud identified other forms of social maladjustment that were not caused by disruptions in the weakening of object-love in the child's very early life but were due to later disturbances in the child's emotional attachments and conflicts during the Oedipal period. Concurring with Melanie Klein, Anna Freud believed these could arise when the child projects his own hostile, aggressive, or anxious urges and fantasies into the external world, even when the child has received adequate parental care. However, in contrast to Klein, Anna Freud stressed the role of infantile sexuality rather than that of infantile aggression in the development of severe social maladjustment or psychopathy. This, she proposed, was due to a complete suppression of phallic masturbation and the consequent flooding of the ego with sexual content and unconscious masturbation fantasies of the pregenital phases, which are then acted out in masochistic, sadistic, scopophilic, or exhibitionistic behaviours (Freud, A., 1947).

Winnicott: The antisocial tendency

The discoveries and writings of the British paediatrician, psychiatrist, and psychoanalyst Donald Winnicott marked a significant contribution to the psychoanalytic understanding of delinquency and criminality. Rooted in his work in the observations and treatment of antisocial children, including those who were evacuated or difficult to billet during the Second World War, he formulated delinquency as a reaction to specific deprivations in infancy and childhood, particularly prolonged separation from the mother.

Winnicott effected a fundamental shift in psychoanalytic thinking about juvenile delinquency in his interpretation of a child's antisocial behaviour as carrying a positive, not negative, value in that it represents a signal of distress and communication for attention and containment. Although Winnicott agreed with Klein that the origin of aggression was innate, he contended that aggressiveness is not solely destructive but inherent in bodily movement as an essential and positive part of normal development. Moreover, play and the use of symbols are essential to contain inner aggression, and when these are not available, playing is replaced by acting out. He believed that the majority of children experience "good enough" mothering, which contains the child's aggressive impulses, but when there is significant frustration or deprivation; for example, a mother who is depressed, or the break-up of the family, pathological aggression may arise, as opposed to the healthy aggression which is integral to the child's growth.

In *Some Psychological Aspects of Juvenile Delinquency* (Winnicott, 1946), Winnicott introduced the idea that delinquency is an indication of hope. Delinquent children and adolescents have suffered deprivation in their home life, which has failed to offer safety and security. Their antisocial behaviour is an unconscious seeking of the good mother, as well as paternal authority to limit their aggressive impulses and regain their primitive love impulses, sense of guilt, and wish to repair. Winnicott elaborated further on the link between delinquent behaviour and hope in two seminal papers: *The Antisocial Tendency* (Winnicott, 2016a [1956]) and *Delinquency as a Sign of Hope* (Winnicott, 2016b [1968]). He stressed that antisocial acts relate to deprivation, not privation: in privation, the child's earliest needs have not been met, ego development is severely affected, and the child is prone to psychosis, whereas in deprivation the child has experienced some degree of adequate care-giving at the beginning of his life, but there is subsequent serious failure in care at a later stage in the infant's development. This then leads to an unconscious yearning in the child for something good that has been lost. Winnicott identified two strands at the roots of the antisocial tendency: stealing and lying, and destructiveness. The first strand may start as greediness, which then progresses to stealing. It is object-seeking not of the actual object that has been stolen but the good experience of the mother that needs to be regained. The second strand, destructiveness, seeks environmental stability which will contain the aggressive impulses.

The antisocial tendency, therefore, is the externalisation of the longing to regain the maternal object and emotional stability; it implies hope, a communication that is seeking a response, and compels the environment to act and attend to the child's management. However, if this disguised cry for help and containment is ignored or the response is solely punitive, the antisocial tendency may harden into real delinquency and form part of the young person's character defences and way of relating to others, which become more difficult to alter. Winnicott believed that the essential component of effective care for delinquency is not psychoanalysis but the provision of environmental care – an alternative to the family in the form of foster parents, therapeutic hostels and detention centres, and residential care.

Bowlby: The affectionless character

John Bowlby was a British psychiatrist and psychoanalyst who was a pioneer in the field of child development and the founder of attachment theory. His paper *Forty-four Juvenile Thieves: Their Characters and Home-Life* (1944) is a foundational work which ushered in his discovery of attachment theory. During the 1930s and 1940s, he worked with maladjusted and delinquent children in schools and state institutions and during the Second World War saw children who had been traumatised by separation and violence. *Forty-four Juvenile Thieves* is his study of 44 delinquent children with a history of stealing, which he compared to a control group referred to the same clinic but with no history of stealing or other forms of delinquency. Bowlby identified an "affectionless" group, who displayed a complete lack of empathy, guilt, or remorse for their actions and responded to neither punishment nor kindness and were not capable of attachment, affection, or loyalty. They were significantly more delinquent than the other thieves and constituted more than half of the more serious and chronic offenders.

Bowlby found a strong link between early attachment disruptions and later delinquency. He considered five causes, but only prolonged separation from the mother or caregiver was strongly associated with persistent offending. The other factors – genetics, ambivalent mothers, hostile fathers, and trauma – were linked to unstable and maladapted children in general but not specifically to delinquency.

Bowlby explored the psychopathology of affectionless children, aligning with Klein and Winnicott in believing that libidinal and aggressive impulses are present from birth, but he emphasised the critical role of the child's relationship with the mother in the first year of life. Like Winnicott, he identified two key expressions of antisocial behaviour: stealing, linked to a craving for maternal love, and aggression, which included revenge. However, unlike Winnicott, who saw these behaviours as communicative, Bowlby focused on the damaging effects of early separation. He argued that separation stimulates libidinal and aggressive instincts and severely inhibits the development of object-love.

In emotionally healthy children, object-love develops through recognising, valuing, and reciprocating the mother's love. This process, via identification and introjection, leads to the formation of the superego, which regulates hostile impulses to preserve attachment to the loved object. Bowlby believed that in affection-less thieves, early separation from the primary caregiver disrupts this process, impeding superego development and the ability to regulate libidinal and aggressive impulses. He suggested their inability to form loving relationships stems from two main causes: a lack of opportunity for attachment during a critical developmental window, and the inhibition of love due to unresolved rage and the phantasies that arise from it.

Bowlby proposed that another factor of importance, particularly in the child who has experienced separation at the slightly later age of 2 or 3, is the determination not to risk being disappointed again. He suggested that the apparent indifference of these children to showing or receiving affection was a policy of self-protection, as if they were saying, "At all costs, let us avoid any risk of allowing our hearts to be broken again" (Bowlby, 1944, p. 124). Bowlby did not refer to these affectionless characters as psychopaths, but nevertheless his paper is credited as being pivotal in describing the lack of attachments that are pathognomonic of a contemporary psychobiological construct of psychopathy, and how the lack of empathy and detachment from others might function as a defence against rejection rather than the expression of an innate incapacity for object relating. This dichotomy will be explored in the following chapters, which examine more recent psychoanalytic conceptualisations of antisocial and psychopathic personalities in the context of empirical research findings from the fields of genetics, neuroscience, and attachment theory.

Part 2

Contemporary perspectives

Chapter 3

Antisocial personality disorder

Aetiological and diagnostic controversies

Diagnostic confusion

Antisocial personality disorder (ASPD) was the first personality disorder to be formally identified as a diagnostic entity and has been the most researched of all the personality disorders. Initially included as sociopathic personality disorder in the first edition of the Diagnostic Statistical Manual, DSM-I (APA, 1952), the disorder was renamed antisocial personality disorder in DSM-II (APA, 1968). Formal criteria for the diagnosis were enumerated in DSM-III, and the disorder is still included as one of ten personality disorders described in DSM-5 (APA, 2013).

However, the DSM-5 criteria for antisocial personality disorder have been criticised for their focus on antisocial behaviour and criminality rather than on the underlying personality structure and interpersonal deficits, as well as diagnostic overlap with other personality disorders and neurodevelopmental disorders and neurodiversity. The inclusion of psychopathy within the overall diagnosis of ASPD has been particularly controversial.

Prior to the introduction of ASPD as a diagnostic category in DSM-III, the terms sociopathy and psychopathy were commonly used interchangeably, despite arising from very different historical traditions. The concept of sociopathy arose from research on social deviancy by the social psychiatrist Lee Robins, who viewed the character disorder through a sociological lens and focussed on the individual's behaviours in relation to their environment and cultures. By contrast, psychopathy reflected a more psychogenic

DOI: 10.4324/9781003559801-6

approach advocated by psychologists such as Robert Hare and others based on Cleckley's criteria for psychopathy, which included problematic personality traits in the interpersonal arena, such as lack of empathy, guilt, and remorse (Houser, 2015). Robins opposed the inclusion of psychopathic traits in the diagnosis of ASPD, and others wanted psychopathy to be listed as a separate personality disorder, but in an effort to prioritise inter-rater reliability rather than validity, the DSM-III criteria were operationalised in behavioural rather than personality terms, and psychopathy was not included as a separate diagnostic entity. More aspects of psychopathy were included in the diagnostic criteria for ASPD in subsequent versions of the DSM, but psychopathy is not individually recognised as a component of the disorder.

This has resulted in the DSM-5 diagnostic category of ASPD encompassing a heterogeneous population which does not distinguish between those individuals with mild, moderate, or severe psychopathy. A substantial body of research has shown that, at most, only one out of three patients with ASPD has severe psychopathy, and this latter group has a significantly poorer treatment prognosis than patients with mild to moderately psychopathic ASPD (Hare, 1991). This suggests that the diagnosis includes separate sub-groups, with different causative factors, trajectories, and responses to treatment.

The dichotomy between psychological versus sociological conceptualisations of ASPD influential in the latter half of the last century has been replaced by a tension between psychogenic and biogenic approaches to antisocial personality disorder. Whilst psychoanalytic theorists have examined the intrapsychic origins of psychopathy with an increasing emphasis on the importance of narcissistic psychopathology and disturbances in early object relations, researchers from other disciplines have become more interested in genetic and neuroscientific empirical research that validates constitutional and organic theories of antisocial and psychopathic character development, identifying neurobiological vulnerabilities that predispose the individual to developing ASPD or psychopathy. It is important to review these findings as these have been integrated into contemporary psychoanalytic theories of ASPD, which address the role of both constitutional and environmental factors in its developmental trajectory and challenge the dichotomy between nature and nurture.

The neurobiology of antisocial personality disorder

There is strong evidence suggesting that ASPD can be understood as a neurodevelopmental disorder with a notable genetic foundation, marked by brain structure and function abnormalities, as well as neurocognitive impairments (Choy & Raine, 2024). Behavioural genetic research has shown that antisocial and psychopathic traits have a moderate to high heritability. Studies of twin pairs have found that up to 75% of the variance in ASPD is attributed to genetic influences. Similarly, numerous twin studies in childhood and adolescence document that psychopathic tendencies or callous unemotional traits, which are thought to be the precursors of psychopathy in adulthood, have a genetic origin (Viding & Larsson, 2010). Studies have also examined candidate genes associated with ASPD, focussing on those involved in the synthesis and regulation of serotonin production, the premise being that low serotonin levels are considered a risk factor for impulsive and aggressive behaviour (Choy & Raine, 2024).

Neuroimaging studies on ASPD have consistently found structural brain abnormalities, particularly in the prefrontal cortex, as well as in the temporal region. Similarly, neuropsychological studies have shown impairments in executive functions such as planning and set shifting, which are consistent with deficits in the frontotemporal regions observed in neuroimaging research. Studies which have examined the overlap between ASPD and psychopathy have suggested that some of these cognitive impairments are specific to ASPD rather than psychopathy (Choy & Raine, 2024).

One of the most consistently replicated findings in the literature on the neurobiology of antisocial behaviour is the functioning of the autonomic nervous system, focusing on key traits such as underarousal and fearlessness. Early research on the underarousal of psychopaths, particularly in response to punishment, revealed reduced peripheral autonomic reactions to aversive stimuli, as measured by skin conductance or galvanic skin response (Hare & Thorvaldson, 1970). This finding has been replicated globally in numerous studies, which show that habitual criminals are chronically underaroused at the cortical level and exhibit abnormal physiological responses to threats (Patrick, 2018). Low cortical arousal has also been associated with children and adolescents displaying callous-unemotional traits (Frick et al., 2003). These children tend to engage in thrill-seeking and fearless behaviours, have difficulty responding to negative stimuli, habituate more easily to the distress of others (Kimonis et al., 2006), and show lower autonomic reactivity to negative emotional stimuli (Blair, 1999). These physiological patterns have been linked to structural and functional brain abnormalities, primarily in the limbic system, especially the amygdala (Yang & Raine, 2018).

These findings have led to the proposition that ASPD is a neurodevelopmental disorder in which genetic factors influence the central nervous system to affect neurocognitive function, and the autonomic nervous system to affect physiological responses, both of which shape the course of an individual developing ASPD (Choy & Raine, 2024).

The role of the environment

It is important to recognise, however, that these neurobiological abnormalities in the brains of individuals with ASPD may not be solely the result of genetic or constitutional factors but could also be the outcome of early environmental experiences that have shaped the structure and function of the developing brain. Numerous studies have found a significant connection between ASPD, including those with high levels of psychopathy, and adverse childhood experiences, such as physical, sexual, and emotional abuse, neglect, harsh parenting, parental mental illness or alcoholism, parental criminality, institutional deprivation, malnutrition, and smoking during pregnancy (e.g., Farrington et al., 2006; Kolla et al., 2013; Dargis et al., 2016; Sevecke et al., 2016).

Behavioural-genetic research has sought to determine the extent to which genetic factors, shared environmental influences, and nonshared environmental factors contribute to variations in psychopathic traits. An increasing body of behavioural-genetic studies has highlighted significant gene-environment interactions, where an individual's genotype affects their level of exposure to environmental risk factors (Hyde et al., 2016).

Primary and secondary psychopathy: The role of anxiety

The presence of anxiety in individuals with ASPD is an important variable in the subtyping of ASPD (De Brito & Hodgins, 2009). Studies of both children and adults suggest that approximately half of individuals with ASPD exhibit anxiety alongside persistent antisocial behaviour, with low levels of callous-unemotional traits as children and low levels of psychopathic traits as adults. This group is more likely to have faced physical abuse during childhood and may turn to violence as a way of coping with underlying emotional conflict and distress. The other half display normal to low levels of anxiety, with varying degrees of psychopathy, including a subgroup with high levels of psychopathy. This latter group tends to show high callous-unemotional traits as children, low anxiety, a greater propensity for predatory violence, and are generally less responsive to treatment.

These findings reflect an earlier typology of psychopathy that had been proposed Benjamin Karpman (1946), an American psychiatrist and proponent of psychoanalysis who distinguished between primary and secondary psychopaths. He proposed that primary psychopaths display an absence of conscience, guilt, attachment, and emotionality, the disorder being primarily constitutional or genetic in aetiology; whereas the antisocial behaviour of secondary psychopaths arises as a response to underlying neurotic conflicts and parental rejection. Laboratory and clinical research have supported this finding: Lykken (1957) differentiated between secondary (anxious) and primary (non-anxious) psychopaths; and Blackburn (1998) demarcated between the anxious, moody, withdrawn psychopath and the hostile, extraverted, and low anxiety psychopath; and other studies followed suit (Gacono & Meloy, 1991). This distinction has been substantiated by more research exploring the relative contributions of biological versus environmental factors in the development of psychopathy.

Marshall and Cooke (1999) found a negative curvilinear relationship between early adverse experiences and psychopathy. They found that for adult psychopaths, as their psychopathic traits increased into the mild to moderate range there was a historical increase in neglect and abuse in their childhood experiences, suggesting that the more severe the psychopathy, the more psychobiologically rooted is its cause.

Attachment

Contemporary psychoanalytic writers, most notably Reid Meloy, Peter Fonagy, and Anthony Bateman, respectively, have sought to integrate this biological and environmental research into a bio-psychogenic model that proposes that although neuroanatomical, neurophysiological, and twin and adoption studies suggest biological and genetic factors are operant in the development of ASPD and psychopathy, early disturbed object relations and other environmental influences are also involved. Attachment theory provides an explanatory aetiological framework that links these biological and environmental influences in the development of ASPD and psychopathy and provides empirical evidence to validate a psychoanalytic object-relational approach to understanding the dynamics of the mind of these individuals.

Stemming from the seminal work of John Bowlby, attachment theory is a body of knowledge concerned with the emotional bonds and interactions between human beings and the psychopathological difficulties which arise when these processes are disturbed (Bowlby, 1969). It proposes a universal need for significant human relationships, which are established at a psychobiological level in early childhood. Attachment theory explores how these relationships are linked to care-giving and care-eliciting behaviours and used to manage fear, vulnerability, and threats of loss across the lifespan. Bowlby's work was influenced by the psychoanalytic theories of Klein and Winnicott, but he was interested in the ethological work of Harry Harlow, who discovered how raising infant monkeys in social isolation had negative effects on their behaviour and interactions with other primates (Harlow et al., 1965).

Attachment is the normal tendency of the infant and young child to seek proximity to its primary caregivers, usually initially the mother, for protection and a feeling of security. This develops in the first year of life to provide a safe haven and secure base for exploration, including exploration of the mind of self and others. Bowlby proposed that the relationship between the mother and baby leads to the latter forming an "internal working model" of that relationship, which influences how the baby deals with stress, anxiety, and loss.

From the outset, attachment theory was concerned with the integration of psychological and biological models of development. Bowlby was interested in how psychological mechanisms affect biological reactions and physiological homeostasis and proposed that attachment is a behavioural system that regulates the effects of external stressors on internal physiological stability by prompting the individual to seek proximity to attachment figures (Bowlby, 1973).

There is convincing evidence suggesting that disrupted attachment experiences play a role in the development of ASPD and psychopathy. Four distinct pathological or insecure attachment styles have been identified and assessed in adults: fearful, preoccupied, disorganised, and dismissive (George et al., 1996). Studies have shown abnormal attachment patterns in forensic patients and prisoners, some of whom were diagnosed with ASPD (van IJzendoorn et al., 1997; Frodi et al., 2001; Levinson & Fonagy, 2004). All these studies reported an over-representation of individuals with dismissing attachment states of mind, where the person is dismissing, derogating, devaluing, or cut-off from attachment relationships and experiences.

A more recent meta-analysis examined the relationship between attachment styles and psychopathic traits, revealing a positive association between psychopathy and insecure attachment styles. The strongest associations were found in forensic and prison populations (van der Zouwen et al., 2018), which aligns with findings that offenders in prisons or secure forensic settings are more likely to report having experienced attachment disruptions, such as separations, abuse, and neglect from early caregivers, compared to the general population (Weeks & Widom, 1998).

This chapter has reviewed the current state of genetic, neuro-biological, and attachment research regarding the aetiology of ASPD. The following two chapters explore contemporary psychoanalytic theories of psychopathy and ASPD respectively, which draw on this empirical research to offer explanatory models encompassing the dynamic nature of the mind as well as its developmental origins.

Chapter 4

Psychopathy

The mind of the psychopath

The American forensic psychologist Reid Meloy has been at the forefront of the psychoanalytic study of psychopathy in recent years. Integrating findings from attachment research, neuroscience, and psychoanalytic object relations theory, he proposes a psychoanalytic theory of the mind of the psychopath in which very early disturbances in separation and identification processes form the bedrock of the primary traits of the psychopath – the lack of attachment, anxiety, and empathy; the domination of egocentricity, grandiosity, and aggression; imitative and dissociative processes, and the lack of moral conscience.

Failures of internalisation

Meloy (1992) proposes that early disruptions in attachment caused by abuse and adversity from primary caregivers subject the infant psychopath to excessively harsh sensory and perceptual experiences. These experiences, in turn, increase the likelihood of developing a narcissistic outer shell that shields the more vulnerable inner self. This concept is akin to Winnicott's (1960) idea of a "false self", which forms prematurely at the cost of the concealed "true self", as well as Cleckley's (1941) "mask of sanity", which hides an underlying core of psychosis.

When consistent and reliable nurturing experiences are lacking, the infant develops an early distrust of the environment, hindering

DOI: 10.4324/9781003559801-7

the internalisation and identification with good objects or experiences essential for healthy development. The prevalence of harsh and harmful objects, combined with a lack of soothing internalisation experiences, leads the child to unconsciously reject the need for nurturing, instead identifying with the harsh, aggressive objects encountered externally, a defence mechanism initially described by Sandor Ferenczi (1994 [1933]) and then Anna Freud (1966 [1936]) as identification with the aggressor. Meloy emphasises that these hostile objects may result from actual abuse by caregivers or may be re-internalised projections of the psychopath's own aggressive impulses in the absence of abuse.

Primitive internalised object relations

Meloy proposes that the psychopathic person's mind operates at a borderline level, as described by Kernberg (1976; 1984). Due to failures in internalising and identifying with whole object relationships, the psychopath's internal world remains two-dimensional, populated by primitive internal objects, or "part-objects". In this internal world, good and bad are not integrated, and self and objects are not fully differentiated as whole, separate, and meaningful entities. The psychopath's relationships with others are driven by narcissism, shaped by a framework of dominance and control, where external objects are seen solely as tools for gratification. These object relationships follow a dyadic structure – predator/prey, dominance/submission – and are upheld through primitive defence mechanisms such as splitting, denial, omnipotence, and projection. This ensures that self-representations are consistently inflated, while object representations are devalued. More mature defence mechanisms, like repression and sublimation, are absent.

Similarly, the psychopath's emotional life is shallow, with a range and depth of feeling like that of a toddler who has yet to learn social interaction. Emotions are primarily focused on the self, with little regard for others as whole beings. These emotions are tied to part-objects and include envy, shame, dysphoria, boredom, frustration, rage, and excitement. Emotional modulation is unstable, with intense emotions that quickly dissipate.

More mature emotions, which are deeper, more complex, and involve an understanding of others as whole individuals and the capacity for secure attachment, such as anger, guilt, fear, sadness, depression, gratitude, remorse, sympathy, and loneliness are absent. Instead, the psychopath's emotional life revolves around envy and shame, two primitive emotions that are perceived as intolerable and thus projected into others, which may trigger violence and the intentional destruction of the object in real life.

Malignant narcissism and the grandiose self

Psychopathy can be viewed as a form of malignant narcissism, a term first coined by the psychoanalyst and Marxist Erich Fromm (1964). Fromm believed that character, including the capacity for envy and destructiveness, evolves from interpersonal and relational experience embedded within the culture and society in which one lives. In contrast to benign narcissism, which arises from a joyful and productive attitude to life, malignant narcissism is derived from what one has; for example, their looks, body, or wealth, rather than what one achieves, and thus limits meaningful connections to others, who are used to inflate and sustain their grandiosity rather than orienting them to the reality of human relationships.

Kernberg elaborated on Fromm's ideas in his description of the grandiose self-structure as a central component of narcissistic personality disorders (Kernberg, 1976). Meloy (1988) goes further in delineating the grandiose self that lies at the core of the psychopath. While the grandiose self is present in all narcissistic personality disorders, it serves as the primary identification in the psychopath. This idealised self-representation confirms the psychopath's identification as a predator who dominates and devalues others as prey, forming the cognitive and emotional core of the self. The grandiose self emerges from the distorted internalisations described earlier, but it remains a fragile structure that must be maintained at all costs to preserve the psychopath's narcissistic equilibrium. This is achieved by constantly reinforcing positive self-representations while projecting all negative objects, affects, and representations onto others.

Unlike individuals with more benign forms of narcissistic personality disturbance, the psychopath cannot maintain the grandiose self merely through fantasy, in which he elevates himself and devalues others. For the grandiose self to be preserved, it requires the actual belittling, defamation, and abuse of others, including through violence. Meloy suggests that this failure of the omnipotent fantasy to contain violence occurs because the psychopath becomes desensitised to his own fantasies, a process exacerbated by chronic low autonomic arousal. As a result, unbearable emotions such as emptiness, shame, and envy surface in consciousness and can only be expelled through the harm of others. By devaluing the object, the psychopath diminishes his envy, as there are no longer any qualities worth possessing, and he reduces his shame, as the object is no longer a source of humiliation.

The psychopathic superego

The hallmark of psychopathy is the absence of guilt, remorse, and moral values – the manifestation of abnormalities in the psychopath's superego. Object relation theorists such as Jacobsen (1964) and Kernberg (1984) suggested that the psychopath's superego is underdeveloped and consists of sadistic precursors – fragments of harsh, persecutory objects that were internalised and identified with during infancy. These aggressive identifications, which replace the normal parental ideals, form a pathological superego that rewards malevolent intentions and destructive behaviours while devaluing positive goals and actions. This accounts for the psychopath's reversal of values or inverse conscience (Svrakic et al., 1991; Richards, 1998). The psychopath assigns negative value to concepts such as attachment, morality, love, and empathy, while giving positive value to aggression, sadism, deception, and greed. Additionally, his identification with badness or evil removes the internal constraints that typically inhibit the gratification of impulses. As the pre-psychopathic child matures, he increasingly aligns with aggressive and destructive peers or mentors outside the family, further solidifying the sadistic superego.

Imitation and simulation

The psychopath's inability to form deep and meaningful connections with others leads him to simulate or imitate others' attitudes and behaviours to blend into society. As described in Chapter 1, the psychoanalyst Greenacre (1958) depicted the psychopath as an imposter, possessing an "as-if" quality and a lack of authenticity. Early unconscious patterns of simulation evolve in later childhood and adolescence into more deliberate imitation of socially acceptable behaviours, aimed at gaining social advantage while simultaneously refining the psychopath's manipulative skills (Glasser, 1986). This explains his ability to exploit, deceive, manipulate, and defraud others while presenting himself as charming, beguiling, and sincere.

Certain individuals may be especially vulnerable to falling victim to the psychopath's deceptions, exploitations, and betrayals (Howell, 2018). Skilled fraudsters or con artists may selectively target victims by identifying subtle narcissistic vulnerabilities – such as a desire for love and acceptance or a yearning for wealth or success, which the psychopath promises to provide. The psychopath may create a false sense of connection with the victim, a process Meloy refers to as "malignant pseudoidentification" (1988), where the psychopath pretends to admire the victim and imitates certain behaviours to create the illusion of a unique bond, which appeals to the victim's narcissism. Symington (1980) further suggests that we are all susceptible to underestimating the psychopath's greed and destructiveness, as acknowledging his sadism forces us to confront our own potential for sadism and destructiveness.

Dissociation

Dissociation is recognised as another foundational psychological process underpinning psychopathy. Dissociation is a defensive process based on the primitive defence mechanism of splitting. In contrast to the horizontal splits in the mind due to repression and negation (Freud, 1938), splitting refers to vertical divisions between otherwise incompatible psychological attitudes, or states of mind, encompassing different goal structures, identity, affects, ideations, subjective experiences, and behavioural manifestations (Kohut, 1971; Kernberg, 1976). Such vertical splits are pathognomonic of borderline ego functioning but are also, according to Meloy (1988), inherent in the psychopathic process. He suggests that psychopaths are particularly prone to dissociative states, such as derealisation and depersonalisation, for several reasons. Firstly, as such states are correlated with high levels of affective or autonomic arousal, due to the psychopath's basal state of chronic peripheral autonomic hypo-arousal, he is prone to seek sensation or high arousal for stimulation. Secondly, dissociative states amplify the psychopath's normal feelings of detachment from other people and his surroundings and enhance his disidentification from external reality. Thirdly, in cases of actual physical violence, the psychopath may use his dissociative state to ensure that his victim remains perceived as a two-dimensional and stereotyped individual without emotional depth, to minimise any meaningful connection between them; and fourthly, memories of dissociative experiences may be used by the psychopath as a rationalisation to avoid responsibility for his actions. For people with borderline personality disorder, dissociative states are experienced as alien or ego-dystonic, but in psychopaths dissociation tends to be ego-syntonic.

Howell (2014) elaborates on Meloy's ideas in tracing the origins of dissociation to childhood trauma by proposing that the psychopath's emulation and mimicking of others' attitudes and behaviours stem from the unconscious simulation and imitation of the behaviour of the psychopath's own childhood abusers, which is internalised as an altered dissociative state. This is a variation of the defence mechanism of identification with the aggressor, in which the abused child, overwhelmed and terrified, enters a trance-like state and identifies with the abuser's wishes and behaviour via mimicry rather than a more purposeful defensive identification. This gives rise to splitting of the psyche into two incompatible dissociative self-states in relation to the abusive caregiver – one of victim, which is attachment oriented, and the other of perpetrator, characterised by aggression. In borderline personality disorder, the mind alternates between these two self-states, which forms the basis of the "stable instability" of the disorder. In contrast, the psychopath's dominant self-state is grandiose, omnipotent, aggressive, and devaluing of others, and any victim-states of fear, shame, humiliation, and vulnerability are rigidly split off and inaccessible or are feigned by the psychopath to exonerate themselves from their crimes. Dissociative processes in psychopathy are deeper, more pervasive and less treatable than those which occur in borderline personalities. The need for attachment itself is dissociated, as awareness of it would be overwhelming and intolerable, making them "outsiders to love" (Howell, 2018).

Psychopathic aggression and violence

Not all psychopaths are violent, but when they are, violence typically does not conflict with their sense of self. The urge for aggression is either immediately acted upon or serves to fuel their grandiose self-image. Due to their lack of attachment, inability to empathise with the victim, and their inverted moral conscience, psychopaths lack the usual internal safeguards that prevent most people from resorting to violence.

The psychoanalyst Mervyn Glasser (1998) introduced a helpful distinction between what he referred to as "self-preservative violence" and "sadomasochistic violence". Both forms of violence stem from an early pathological relationship with the mother, where aggression is unconsciously employed to create distance and separation from an overpowering maternal figure.

Self-preservative violence is a basic, instinctive reaction triggered by any perceived threat to one's physical or psychological self. These threats can include attacks on self-esteem, frustration, humiliation, or insults to ideals that the person values. These threats may also be internal, such as feeling attacked by a sadistic superego or fearing a loss of identity due to feelings of disintegration and confusion, which may occur in psychotic disorders. The violent response in self-preservative violence is primal, immediate, and focused on eliminating the source of the perceived danger.

In contrast, sadomasochistic violence is not an instant reaction but is premeditated and strategically executed to fulfil violent intentions, such as torturing and controlling victims. A key difference between the two types of violence lies in their relationship to the object or victim. In self-preservative violence, the target is seen solely as an immediate threat, with no personal significance beyond that. The victim's emotional responses or identity as a whole person is irrelevant – the focus is simply on eliminating the perceived danger. In sadomasochistic violence, the victim's reactions are essential: the victim must be seen to suffer, and to achieve this, they must be kept alive. Sadomasochistic violence also involves pleasure, which distinguishes it from self-preservative violence, where anxiety is always present. Glasser provides a clear example of the difference between the two types of violence: a soldier who kills an enemy in battle, believing it necessary to protect himself from being killed, is engaging in self-preservative violence. However, a soldier who captures an enemy and tortures them to make them suffer is enacting sadomasochistic violence.

Although these might seem to be two very different forms of violence, Glasser saw these as the two poles on a continuum of violent behaviours, in which the appreciation of the object as a person to be controlled and manipulated decreases as one moves from the sexual to overtly violent, and that sadomasochistic violence can be seen as a more mature, albeit pathological, defence against the more primitive anxiety-driven self-preservative violence.

While Glasser was developing his ideas on self-preservative and sadistic aggression with colleagues at the Portman Clinic, Meloy (1988; 1992; 2006) applied object relations theory and attachment theory to create a bimodal model of violence, which has its roots in animal physiology research from half a century earlier. Meloy, along with other researchers including Eichelman (1988), McEllistrem (2004), and Siegel and Victoroff (2009), expanded on the physiological, pharmacological, and forensic differences between two psychobiologically distinct types of violence: "affective" and "predatory". Affective aggression, sometimes referred to as emotional or reactive aggression, aligns with Glasser's self-preservative aggression. This type of violence is characterised by high levels of sympathetic arousal and intense emotion (usually anger or fear) and occurs as a response to an immediate threat.

Predatory violence, also known as instrumental violence, is similar to Glasser's concept of sadomasochistic violence. It is marked by a lack of emotion, careful planning, and preparation. This type of violence is common among psychopaths and is facilitated by their diminished autonomic arousal, meaning they do not consciously experience anxiety or fear, which allows them to carry out predatory actions without inhibition. Predatory violence can be intensified using psychostimulants like cocaine, which amplify the grandiose self-image and increase the drive for violent behaviour to sustain it. The execution of homicides, sexual homicides, and serial killings – crimes committed by a minority of psychopaths – often involve predatory violence. These acts are typically preceded by rehearsal fantasies of grandiosity and omnipotence, as well as private rituals where the planned violence is enacted in less extreme forms. Psychopathic offenders are more likely than other criminals to engage in both affective and predatory violence (Cornell et al., 1996; Woodworth & Porter, 2002).

Meloy cites evidence from empirical research to argue that different neurophysiological pathways underpin these two different forms of violence, which are not linked, as Glasser suggests, with his continuum, and that psychopathic aggression or violence is not a defence against underlying anxiety or other painful affects. However, other psychoanalytic writers, such as the American psychiatrist James Gilligan (1996), see psychopathy as a defensive structure erected in reaction to early childhood trauma and emphasise the role of shame and humiliation in precipitating all forms of violence. Drawing on his work with high-security inmates in the American penal system, Gilligan found that the offenders' early experiences of being rejected, ostracised, abused, or made to feel as if they did not exist predisposed them as adults to be sensitised to feeling ostracised, bullied, or ignored, leading to unbearable feelings of shame and humiliation which needed to be expelled by violent means. Gilligan believes that shame is integral to all violent acts. This may be more evident in self-preservative or affective violence, where the painful affect is consciously felt and must be defended against but may also be present in sadomasochistic or psychopathic violence, where early experiences of shame have been completely dissociated, so that any hint of humiliation is immediately denied and projected via the violent destruction of others. Howell (2018) stresses that if the psychopath is in touch with these shame states, this would be akin to being psychically annihilated, as in childhood, all over again.

This chapter has focussed on current psychoanalytic insights and conceptualisations of psychopathy, rather than consideration of the broader psychiatric diagnosis of antisocial personality disorder, which includes antisocial individuals who are not psychopathic. The next chapter will examine this disorder through the lens of mentalisation, arguably the most prominent model of human relating and modality of treatment that has emerged from the psychoanalytic stable in recent years.

Chapter 5

Mentalisation and antisocial personality disorder

The developmental origins of mentalising

Mentalisation is a concept describing a social cognition that has been elaborated on and refined by the clinical psychologist and psychoanalyst Peter Fonagy and his colleagues over the past 25 years from its roots in psychoanalytic theory and attachment theory within the crucible of developmental psychopathology. Mentalisation develops within a relational context – importantly, but not exclusively, in the early attachment relationships with primary caregivers – which is necessary for human beings to operate within a social world and to meaningfully relate to others. In its exploration of psychological processes, the theory of mentalisation has had wide-reaching influence in clinical practice, particularly in the understanding of personality disorders and other mental disorders and the development of tailored psychological treatments for these conditions; and its scientific credentials continue to be affirmed by new research findings in developmental psychology, psychopathology, and neuroscience.

Mentalisation is the capacity to reflect on and to think about mental states, including thoughts, beliefs, desires, and affects, to be able to distinguish one's own mental states from others, and to be able to interpret the actions and behaviour of oneself and others as meaningful and based on intentional mental states (Bateman & Fonagy, 2019). The normal development of mentalisation is dependent on the intersubjective process of emerging psychological awareness between the child and his primary caregivers in the

DOI: 10.4324/9781003559801-8

context of a secure attachment. The child becomes increasingly aware of his own mind through his growing awareness of the mind of his mother, or trusted other, through her capacity to demonstrate to him, via her empathic mirroring, that she experiences him as a separate person with his own distinct intentions, beliefs, and desires. The quality of affective mirroring, particularly the capacity for contingent emotional responsiveness by the caregiver, is critical for the normal development of affect regulation, impulse control, attentional mechanisms, and mentalisation. Disruptions in attachment, including abuse and trauma, combined with constitutional vulnerabilities, can lead to impairments in the capacity for mentalisation. This can lead to character pathology in adulthood, such as in borderline personality disorder (BPD) and ASPD, in which the capacity for mentalisation is fragile and developmentally earlier modes of thinking about subjective experience are triggered in the context of emotionally intense attachment relationships. As described in Chapter 3, many studies indicate that disrupted attachment experiences play a role in the development of psychopathy and ASPD. ASPD can therefore be conceptualised as a disorder of mentalising and attachment in which genetic precursors interact with early environmental adversity to result in abnormal personality development, particularly in the areas of emotional regulation, impulse control, and the ability to mentalise.

Pre-mentalising modes

Fonagy and colleagues have identified several primitive modes of thinking that predate the emergence of mentalising and are present in normal early childhood development but are more likely to persist and re-emerge in people with certain personality disorders, in particular BPD and ASPD, when the attachment system is reactivated and mentalising fails. These pre-mentalistic or non-mentalising modes of organising subjective experience include what they call "psychic equivalence", "pretend mode", and "teleological thinking".

Psychic equivalence is a state of concrete thinking in which internal and external reality are experienced as isomorphic, thoughts are felt to be real, there is no tolerance of differing points of view, doubt is suspended, and thoughts cannot be symbolised.

In extreme cases, a disturbed subjective state of mind is experienced as pseudo-psychotic symptoms, or as flashbacks in post-traumatic stress disorder.

In pretend mode, sometimes referred to as "hypermentalising" or "pseudomentalising", thoughts and feelings are dissociated from reality to the point of meaninglessness, so that a person may appear to be talking about important internal experiences, but these are disconnected from any meaningful context. The person shows cognitive understanding of mental states but little affective understanding. In states of extreme pretend mode, the person may experience states of dissociation or derealisation.

Teleological mode refers to a mode of thinking in which the motivations of others are interpreted according to the presence of physical actions and where changes in mental states are only felt to be real when confirmed by physically observable action. Teleological mode may be expressed in dramatic or destructive actions; for example, behaviours such as self-harm or violence, which are felt to be the only method of communicating with others.

The alien self

Early traumatic experiences can also lead to impairments in the development of a stable sense of self. The mother (or alternative caregiver) who is not attuned to her baby's experience will provide inadequate mirroring of the infant's behaviour, so that the child is unable to develop a representation of his own experience and instead internalises the image of the caregiver. Where the primary caregiver has been neglectful or frankly malevolent towards the child, this internalised representation will be experienced as foreign or bad and will never be fully integrated into his overall schema of self-representations. Fonagy and colleagues have called this discontinuity within the self the "alien self" and suggest that this internalised self-representation is subject to the pressure of projection into others to maintain the illusion of a self that does not contain unacceptable aspects. This results in a disorganised self-structure involving the continual re-externalisation of intolerably painful self-states, particularly negative affects associated with vulnerability, shame, and humiliation.

Dimensions of mentalising

Mentalising is a multi-dimensional construct containing several underlying polarities which are most likely related to relatively distinct neural systems (Bateman & Fonagy, 2019). Mentalising can be considered as four intersecting dimensions or functional polarities: automatic/controlled (or implicit/explicit); internally/externally based; self/other orientated; and cognitive/affective process. Successful mentalising involves integrating all of these dimensions into a coherent whole: this is difficult for all of us, but people with personality pathology may show particular impairments in one or more of these polarities.

The automatic (implicit) and controlled (explicit) dimension is the most fundamental polarity underlying mentalising. Implicit mentalising is a non-conscious, non-reflexive, procedural function that requires little effort or attention, whereas explicit mentalising is a much slower process which is more conscious, usually verbal, and requires effort, attention, and reflection. In our normal daily interactions and interpersonal situations, we predominantly use implicit mentalising, especially in the context of secure attachment relationships, and it is only when something unexpected or unusual occurs that we may need to consciously slow down, reflect, and explicitly think about what has happened.

The external/internal mentalising dimension refers to the target of mentalising. Internal mentalising is a focus on one's own or others' internal states – i.e., their thoughts, feelings, intentions, and desires; external mentalising implies a reliance on the external world or external features of others such as facial expression and non-verbal behaviours in interpreting intentions and making sense of interpersonal situations.

The external/internal mentalising dimension differs from the self/other mentalising dimension, which refers to the object of focus of mentalising (i.e., the self or others). Impairments in mentalising may manifest similarly in both self and others (e.g., they may be primarily internally oriented in both) or there may be marked imbalances in mentalising about the self and others. For example, the mentalising of patients with narcissistic personality disorder is primarily focused on the self, whereas people with antisocial and psychopathic traits may be expert at reading other people's internal states – at least at a cognitive level – with little understanding of their own.

The final dimension of mentalising relates to cognitive and affective processing. Cognitive processing encompasses belief-desire reasoning and perspective taking, whereas affective processing includes emotional empathy, subjective self-experience, and mentalised affectivity. Full mentalising requires the integration of both cognitive and affective processes.

Imbalances within these dimensions may generate non-mentalising modes of subjectivity. In psychic equivalence, there is dominance of affect over cognition. In pretend mode, explicit mentalising is lost, and the person is dominated by implicit mentalising with little capacity for reflection. Teleological mode occurs where there is too much focus on external events to the neglect of internal experience.

Mentalising in Antisocial Personality Disorder

Although individuals with ASPD show difficulties in mentalising, their incapacity to mentalise is not absolute but is exhibited in specific imbalances in the dimensions of mentalising and associated subjective pre-mentalising states of mind.

People with ASPD are, by definition, antisocial but are paradoxically dependent on their relationships with others into whom they can project alien aspects of themselves to stabilise their minds and feel a sense of self-coherence. Relationships in individuals with ASPD tend to be rigid, hierarchical, and controlling, as exemplified in dismissive attitudes towards women, who are viewed as inferior, or in the "gang culture" of organised crime. Notions of recognition and respect, often enshrined in an unspoken code of conduct, assume a special importance in their interpersonal relationships, as this affirms and validates the person's fragile sense of self. If, however, such relationships are challenged by the other person refusing to be the recipient of their malign projections; for example, the subjugated wife who talks back to her abusive husband, the return of the alien self and unbearable feelings of shame and humiliation threaten the person's fragile stability of mind, which may trigger violence in an attempt to regain control and a sense of integrity.

Individuals with ASPD show imbalances in the dimensions of mentalising (Bateman et al., 2019). They find it difficult to explicitly mentalise themselves and others due to their lack of interest in what other people think and feel. They therefore tend to overuse automatic mentalising, which is compromised because their assumptions about themselves and others are not informed or challenged. In relation to the cognitive-affective dimension of mentalising, they may demonstrate a good cognitive understanding of mental states but lack a capacity to connect with the affective core of others. This is evident in the absence of compassion or empathy for others. Moreover, their cognitive capacities become distorted in self-serving ways such that they become convinced of their own convictions, rather than being able to consider and incorporate the views of others. These deficits within the cognitive-affective axis are reflected in asymmetry and fixations at one or other poles of the self-other axis of mentalising. They fail to see aspects of themselves in the other person, and vice versa, which facilitates their disregard for the rights of others and permits antisocial and violent behaviour, as their experience of the other person's reaction and feelings do not constrain them. Their excessive focus on either self or other means that their relationships tend to be one-sided, and their social interaction is impaired. In general, individuals with ASPD find it difficult to differentiate internal from external states and to reflect on their own internal states and explore their current experiences. They also tend to misinterpret other people's expressed facial or other external emotions, which results in difficulties and delays in gaining information about others' mental states, particularly in relation to affect.

These disparities in the dimensions of mentalising in people with ASPD are reflected in a shift to pre-mentalising ways of thinking. Mentalising that is too focused on external cues, coupled with difficulties in reflection on mental states, predisposes an individual to a psychic equivalence mode where others' motives and intentions are interpreted, often in a paranoid way, based on external appearance, which can lead to problems in social interactions. For example, the way another person uses eye contact with the individual with ASPD may be perceived as malevolent or disrespectful, which may result in conflict.

The imbalance in individuals with ASPD between mentalising the self and mentalising others, with excessive focus on one at the expense of the other, lends itself to pretend mode, where thoughts and feelings become dissociated and dehumanised, such that meaningful connections with others are not possible. The person is unable to resonate with emotional states that include recognition and appreciation of others, such as love, guilt, or fear, which would normally inhibit someone from being violent. As described in Chapter 4, people with psychopathy and ASPD are prone to experiencing dissociative states of derealisation and depersonalisation, which may be understood as severe conditions of pretend mode.

Teleological mode tends to drive motivation for action for people with ASPD. In this mindset, the person's experience is only considered valid only when its consequences are clearly visible and tangible. Great emphasis is placed on the importance of appearance and "face"; for example, a person is considered successful if observed to be wearing expensive clothes or owning a luxury car. Similarly, loyalty to the gang is demonstrated by observable acts of physical violence or retribution.

Individuals with ASPD who are psychopathic may show some enhanced areas of mentalisation; for example, in their ability to deceive and exploit others, which necessitates an ability to understand the mind of the other to predict what he will and will not believe (Fonagy & Bateman, 2006). However, they caution that this apparently highly tuned capacity to mentalise is very restricted and rarely generalisable to complex interpersonal situations. This substantiates Baron-Cohen's salient description of psychopathy as exemplifying a partial but fundamental impairment of mentalising – i.e., mindreading without empathising (Baron-Cohen, 2005).

Violence in ASPD

Violence can be understood in relation to these primitive modes of thinking. Bateman and Fonagy (2008) propose that reactive or affective violence arises where there is a failure or inhibition of the capacity for mentalisation. The person with ASPD experiences psychic stability so long as projection of the alien self remains successful, but when this fails, pre-mentalistic types of thinking emerge, especially teleological thinking. A person with a limited capacity to mentalise is not able to manage negative emotions such as normal anger, hatred, and wishes to hurt but instead may become highly aroused very quickly and experience themselves as unable to think and overwhelmed with negative affects. As described by Gilligan (1996), the person with ASPD, who is already highly sensitive to threats to his self-worth or "respect", cannot tolerate internal emotional states of shame and humiliation, which are experienced as threatening his very psychic survival. These unbearable feelings cannot be managed by representational means within his mind but are experienced very concretely in psychic equivalence mode as feelings that he needs to expel in violent action or teleologically. The expression of aggression is further potentiated by the reduced capacity of the individual to mentalise – if he is unable to see others as having mental states as different from himself, this will reduce the inhibition of his aggression and violence towards others as he is unable to empathise or appreciate another person's suffering. Moreover, the onset of pretend mode creates an illusory sense of safety in which the violent person is detached from reality and hence the danger and consequences of his actions.

There is some evidence that the propensity for more instrumental or psychopathic, rather than reactive, violence may also be impacted by the capacity for mentalisation. Taubner et al. (2012), in a study of adolescents, found that the ability to mentalise moderated the relationship between psychopathic traits and psychopathy. In this study, individuals with psychopathic traits who had a higher ability to mentalise showed less proactive aggression than those with a lower capacity for mentalisation. Mentalisation therefore protects against violence, and individuals whose capacity for mentalisation is reduced are more likely to be violent.

Epistemic trust

Fonagy and colleagues have introduced the concept of *epistemic trust* into the mentalising framework to reconceptualise personality disorders (Fonagy et al., 2015). Epistemic trust refers to a uniquely human, evolutionary capacity for recognising communication as trustworthy and relevant, facilitating the transfer of social and cultural knowledge. Infants are especially attuned to *ostensive cues* – signals like eye contact, turn-taking, and "motherese" – which indicate that the caregiver sees them as intentional beings. This fosters openness to learning and the development of agency, where the caregiver is experienced as a reliable source of knowledge. As the child grows up, this trust is extended to other significant people and eventually generalises to personal and social relationships so that the adult is open to receiving new information from others, which is necessary to effectively navigate the social world.

Securely attached children are more likely to develop epistemic trust. In contrast, those exposed to trauma, neglect, or abuse often develop "epistemic mistrust", viewing others' communications with suspicion. This can result in "epistemic hypervigilance", where others' intentions are overinterpreted, leading to anxiety, rigid thinking, and interpersonal difficulties. Such individuals may crave validation yet reject it, reinforcing a cycle of mistrust and social alienation.

From the perspective of epistemic trust, personality disorders may be understood as arising from the person being unable to access cultural communication that is relevant to the self from the social context. This is at variance with traditional models of personality disorder, which emphasise the abnormality of the person's character – i.e., the disorder of their personality; by contrast, within the model of epistemic trust, personality disorder is conceptualised as a failure of communication in which learning from others is disordered. This accounts for the clinical experience of such patients as being difficult to engage in treatment or "hard to reach", which is a particular characteristic of many individuals with a diagnosis of ASPD. Therapeutic strategies to address this, as well as other principles of assessment and treatment for patients with ASPD, will be considered in the next chapter.

Part 3

Clinical considerations

Chapter 6

General principles of assessment and treatment

Therapeutic pessimism

Many psychiatrists and other professionals within health and criminal justice have long held beliefs that patients with ASPD, and particularly those with psychopathy, are untreatable. Such therapeutic pessimism has been based on a lack of empirical evidence for the efficacy of any specific treatment intervention, as well as the risks such patients pose, including violence, substance misuse, and boundary violations. Mental health services specifically for the treatment of ASPD are scarce; individuals often, especially in mid-life, present to health services with anxiety or depression, but may be denied treatment when the diagnosis of ASPD is made. However, the refusal to treat individuals with ASPD may also be explained by unacknowledged counter-transferential responses in professionals, which unconsciously defend against the powerful and uncomfortable feelings evoked by such patients, many of whom do not willingly accept treatment and lead clinicians to feel angry, despondent, or doubting their own professional capacities.

A psychoanalytically-informed framework

Although only a minority of people with a diagnosis of ASPD may be suitable for formal psychological therapy, a psycho-analytically-informed framework is useful in structuring and guiding the overall management of such individuals within the

DOI: 10.4324/9781003559801-10

setting in which they are seen. For offenders with ASPD, the stated aims of management and treatment may differ between professionals involved, reflecting inherent conflict and ambiguity between the purpose and aims of different agencies in the criminal justice and health systems. These pivot around dichotomies between punishment versus rehabilitation; and reducing the offender's risk to the public versus improving his health and wellbeing. A psychoanalytic approach, with its emphasis on the unconscious determinants of behaviour, is well placed to understand and identify unconscious conflicts, tolerate uncertainty, and negotiate the complex dynamics that occur between the offender, the professionals involved, and the organisations in which the work takes place. Such a framework considers: 1) assessment of risk, not only of the individual patient but also of the setting in which treatment is delivered, and how the emotional or countertransference responses of professionals influence risk; 2) assessment of the patient to ascertain the severity of psychopathy and which personality traits and characteristics may be amenable to treatment depending on available resources; 3) general principles of treatment, including how to engage the patient in a therapeutic process; and 4) specific therapeutic approaches which encompass both the mode of delivery, which may be individual, group, or occasionally family therapy, and the therapeutic interventions used in treatment, including those which are rooted in a psychoanalytic or psychodynamic model. Each of these will be considered in turn.

Risk assessment

A psychoanalytic approach to risk assessment enhances rather than replaces more conventional methods of evaluation of patients or offenders with ASPD. Such an approach highlights how countertransference reactions, changes in the therapeutic frame, the type of violence, and the unconscious meaning of the violent act can affect both the risk of the antisocial patient and the risk prediction of professionals.

Countertransference and risk assessment

There are many risk assessment instruments used in forensic settings that utilise a combination of actuarial factors and structured clinical judgement, such as the Psychopathy Checklist Revised (PCL-R) (Hare, 2003), the Violence Risk Appraisal Guide-Revised (VRAG) (Rice et al., 2013), and the Historical Clinical Risk Management-20 Version 3 (HCR-20) (Douglas et al., 2013) to evaluate a patient's or offender's risk of violence to others. However, these measures do not consider the influence of the assessor's unconscious subjective responses, or countertransference, on their judgement of risk. Blumenthal et al. (2010) showed that the emotional responses of experienced professionals who are well trained in structured and actuarial risk assessment impacted their predication of risk, in that they often unconsciously ignored actuarial risk factors, such as the presence of previous violence or offending, and over-estimated or underestimated the patient's risk according to their subjective judgement or countertransference.

Professionals, particularly those working in the criminal justice system, are often reluctant to admit to experiencing any feelings towards their clients, let alone the disturbing emotional responses that are inevitably evoked by patients with severe antisocial psychopathology. However, if these reactions are not acknowledged and explored, the professional is more likely to act in inappropriate ways. Common countertransference reactions towards offender patients include moral outrage and beliefs that the person is untreatable; feelings of hopelessness and guilt when change does not occur; disgust; excessive fear and its counterpart, the denial of real dangerousness; devaluation and loss of professional identity; excessively punitive and sadistic responses; and sexual excitement, which is rarely admitted or spoken about but can lead to boundary violations (Meloy & Yakeley, 2013).

Emotional responses like disgust may often be felt more in the body than the mind. In a study of 584 professionals, Meloy and Meloy (2003) found that over 75% who interviewed adult psychopaths reported strong physical reactions, such as chills, numbness, stomach tension, or rapid heartbeat, linked to autonomic nervous system activation. These visceral, instinctive responses may serve as primitive danger signals, potentially alerting professionals to elevated risk in their interactions.

Insufficient analysis of countertransference responses can lead to flawed risk assessments, potentially increasing the actual risk. For example, patients' behaviours may trigger feelings of condemnation, fear, or disgust, prompting professionals to respond with punitive or sadistic actions. This can result in an overestimation of risk and the implementation of inappropriate measures, such as extended incarceration or physical restraint. The patient's resulting anger and sense of being mistreated can, in turn, heighten the likelihood of dangerous behaviour.

Other offenders might evoke sympathy and portray themselves as innocent victims, absolving themselves of responsibility for their actions. This can appeal to a clinician's "rescue fantasies", where they wish to help patients they believe have been misunderstood or mistreated by other professionals, potentially leading to an underestimation of the risk involved.

Countertransference responses will vary between professionals, according to their own unconscious object relations and valency for being the recipient of projections of the patient or offender. Thus, a whole picture of the patient's internal world can only be achieved by examining and integrating the different countertransference experiences between different members of the team. If these emotional responses remain unacknowledged and unexplored, they may impact team and institutional dynamics and negatively influence the culture and functioning of the whole organisation which provides the setting in which the antisocial person is seen.

The setting

In all institutional, residential, or community settings where ASPD patients or offenders are managed or treated, considerations of risk, containment, and the communication of information are essential and can be thought about from a psychoanalytic perspective. The setting, whether it be a high-, medium-, or low-security in-patient ward, a prison, or the community, must be secure enough to ensure the safety of both patients and staff before treatment planning can begin.

For antisocial patients, creating a containing therapeutic environment is crucial for effective treatment and ongoing risk management. Risk can only be safely managed when the anxieties of the patients, staff, and the institution are properly contained. However, as described above, due to the disturbing nature of their criminal activities and offending behaviours, forensic patients and offenders may evoke extreme emotional reactions in staff tasked with their management or care. Furthermore, these patients' dismissing and rejecting stance towards relationships, especially those associated with care, which may be conceptualised as re-enactments of their earlier experiences of abusive or neglectful caregivers, may alienate and provoke unconscious retaliatory reactions from clinical and managerial staff. This may lead to the enforcement of even stricter and more punitive measures, or alternatively professionals become complicit, contributing to a dangerously permissive and distorted environment, which mirrors the trauma, lack of boundaries, and unpredictability of their childhood experiences. Thus, the staff group or forensic institution in its entirety may behave in ways, and employ pathological collective defence mechanisms, which reflect the problematic dynamics of the patients' or offenders' families of origin. This re-triggers unbearable emotions of anxiety, shame, and humiliation, with their concomitant aggressive defensive responses, creating a vicious cycle of enactment and re-enactment reverberating between patients, staff, and institution.

Thus, a containing environment is achieved not only by establishing consistent, well-defined, and controlled external structures but also by recognising the unconscious interactions between patients, professionals, and the wider organisation. Such a focus on the relationships between patients or offenders and staff has been referred to as "relational security". However, this needs constantly attending to through staff training, supervision, and support to prevent the high rates of staff turnover, absenteeism, boundary violations, and burnout common in forensic settings. Staff can be supported through psychoanalytically-informed multidisciplinary case discussions and reflective practice groups to explore their countertransference responses, address and manage the anxieties triggered within them, and understand how patients' psychopathologies might be reflected within the institution and lead to pathological team dynamics and staff fragmentation which can paralyse therapeutic efforts. This is exemplified in the following account of a reflective practice group.

Fortnightly reflective practice sessions were delivered by a forensic psychotherapist to a multidisciplinary team employed by the probation service to provide support and treatment for offenders with ASPD. The team was comprised of probation officers, psychologists, mental health practitioners, an assistant psychologist, a housing officer, and the team administrator. The forensic psychotherapist had cancelled the previous session at short notice due to her being unwell. In this session, one of the female psychologists, who was visibly pregnant, wanted to talk about a man who had been referred for psychological work as there were differences of opinion in the team regarding his diagnosis. He evoked strong reactions from professionals due the violent nature of his index offence, in which he had stalked an ex-girlfriend then held her hostage in his flat and raped her. He had recently been released after serving a long prison sentence but was at risk of being evicted from his hostel due to his argumentative behaviour. The psychologist stated that she was very worried about this man's risk to others. He appeared to show no remorse for his offences, despite having completed a sex offender treatment programme whilst in custody and shared no insight into his aggressive behaviour with hostel staff, whom he accused of provoking him, and he exhibited a degree of entitlement in demanding that he was rehoused in a nicer environment. The psychologist felt hemmed in by his incessant demands and thought his attitude towards others indicated a level of psychopathy that was not amenable to treatment. Moreover, she was both worried about and frustrated with his (female) probation officer, who was not present at this session nor answering her emails and wondered whether the probation officer was robust enough to manage him.

Another probation officer, a man, said he disagreed with the psychologist regarding her assessment of the offender. He drew attention to a psychiatric report conducted a few years previously which suggested that he had autistic traits, and he wondered whether this man's difficulties in interpersonal relationships were due to autism, not psychopathy. He added that he had not experienced him as risky but as a child wanting attention and felt that his difficulties in coping in the community were due to a lack of family support and having become institutionalised in prison. The (male) housing officer agreed, saying that he felt quite protective towards him and wanted to ensure that he did not become homeless and be recalled to custody. The probation officer added that he thought his colleague, the offender's probation officer, was not replying to emails due to the current pressures of working in the criminal justice system, which was understaffed and underfunded, rather than her inability to manage this particular client.

The psychologist said she now felt even more infuriated and that her professional expertise was being undermined in the suggestion that the man's diagnosis was uncertain. Moreover, the NHS was also under financial pressure, and there were staff shortages, but she had the courtesy to answer emails. Another psychologist, an older man, commented in a rather intellectual manner that it was interesting how this man's lack of empathy illustrated the diagnostic overlap and confusion between autism, psychopathy, and narcissistic personality disorder. The assistant psychologist, a young woman, interjected that she had been asked to meet with him to carry out some psychometric testing but felt uncomfortable as he had asked her how old she was and that he liked what she was wearing. The administrator, an older woman, said that because she wasn't a clinician she couldn't comment on his diagnosis but had seen him in the office and he looked broken, as if he'd been released back into a world that had changed beyond his recognition and that he was doing all he could to ensure he was sent back to jail.

The forensic psychotherapist eventually commented that there seemed to be some tensions within the team in relation to their client, which perhaps could give them an insight into his internal world but also how his behaviour opened up fault lines in relation to gender and profession and the level of experience amongst themselves within an already splintered system. She said on the one hand there seemed to be a split, reflecting a victim/perpetrator dynamic between the younger women in the team, the psychologist, and assistant psychologist, who felt intimidated by this man whose controlling and inappropriate behaviour towards them paralleled his index offence of holding a woman hostage; and on the other hand, the older members present today, who appeared to be more in touch with the offender's vulnerability, the anxiety, and confusion that presumably was concealed and defended against by his aggressive behaviour. This dichotomy was reflected in confusion about robustness and fragility – was the client so powerful and anxiety-provoking that professionals became overwhelmed and went off sick (reminding them that she also had been ill two weeks ago) or was he too damaged to survive in a system that was itself broken and induced staff burnout? This also highlighted splits between health and criminal justice professionals and a rivalry as to which setting was the hardest in which to work. She added that perhaps the debate about his diagnosis served as a collective defence against really being in touch with intolerable anxieties, projected by the patient into those around him, that were so difficult contain – the horror of his crime, the barrenness of his internal world, and the desperateness of his plight. Could the team come together to support each other in such difficult work? The female psychologist then apologised for her angry outburst, saying she felt more vulnerable being pregnant and that perhaps this man's attacks on women stemmed from not having had the maternal care he deserved.

Degree of psychopathy and type of violence

As explored in Chapter 4, not all individuals with antisocial personality disorder are psychopathic, but those with severe psychopathy not only pose more serious risk of harm to others but also have a significantly poorer treatment prognosis than patients with mild to moderately psychopathic traits. The degree of psychopathy should therefore be evaluated with an instrument such as the PCL-R.

When considering risk, it is also crucial to examine the different forms of violence a person may engage in. Revisiting Glasser's distinction between self-preservative and sadomasochistic violence, self-preservative (affective) violence is a reaction to an immediate threat, where the individual experiences anxiety and operates in fight-or-flight mode. This type of violence is more primitive and dangerous, but if the perceived threat to the self is understood, future triggers can potentially be anticipated. In contrast, sadomasochistic (predatory) violence, while often posing a less immediate risk due to its planned nature (such as grooming the victim), can be harder for the perpetrator to relinquish since it is a source of pleasure.

Meaning of the violent act in the dynamic relationship between the offender and others

To assess risk, it is also important to understand the meaning of the person's antisocial behaviour in relation to their history and current relationships. Psychoanalytically, violence is not a senseless act but represents a form of acting out, a communication with unconscious meaning. In his seminal paper *Remembering, repeating and working through,* Freud says,

> ... the patient does not remember anything of what he has forgotten and repressed, but acts it out. He reproduces it not as a memory, but as an action: he repeats it, without, of course, knowing that he is repeating it. For instance, the patient does not say that he remembers that he used to be defiant and critical towards his parents' authority; instead, he behaves that way to the doctor.
>
> (Freud, 1914, p. 150)

Thus, an apparently unprovoked and inexplicable attack on a female stranger might partly reflect the patient's unconscious anger towards his mother for ignoring the abuse he suffered from his stepfather during childhood. Consciously, the patient may insist that he adores his mother and views her as a victim of domestic violence. However, this patient might be especially sensitive to having a female therapist, whom he may initially idealise but later react to with aggression if he feels rejected or ignored, such as when sessions are cancelled.

Risk assessment and management should therefore include an understanding of how the antisocial person experiences and interacts with others, particularly in how this relates to their early, significant object relationships. This can be further explored in the transference dynamics that will inevitably emerge between the individual and the professionals involved in his care, as the offender will unconsciously repeat his usual patterns of interaction with those treating him, just as he does in all his relationships. Examining these relationships in the context of the offender's early history and criminal behaviour may facilitate a more accurate assessment of the potential risk he may pose.

Changes in the therapeutic frame

Any change or violation in this containment or therapeutic frame, on the part of the offender or therapist, however seemingly insignificant, may indicate increased risk; for example, breaks in therapy or a change of mental health worker. The erratic attendance of the patients and their conscious denial of attachment needs and rejection of treatment may impede clinicians' awareness of the impact of interruptions in therapy, which may trigger intense feelings of loss and rejection in the patient who has unconsciously become dependent on the therapist, key worker, or even institution. Where such feelings are not acceptable in consciousness they may be acted out in violence. When considering risk assessment and psychotherapeutic treatment, it is therefore important to understand such anxieties in the patient and be alert to their appearance in the transference. Ambivalent feelings in relation to the ending of therapy should also be expected and explored, if possible, to avert premature drop-out.

Risk formulation

It should be emphasised that current approaches to risk assessment and management suggest that the focus should shift away from prediction, which is often unreliable, towards developing a formulation of risk. This involves asking in what circumstances the risk of specific behaviours might increase for a particular individual and understanding why. By exploring the unconscious meaning of the antisocial act, it becomes possible to anticipate when the offender might pose a danger again. The formulation helps guide clinical decision-making, determining whether and under what conditions a psychological intervention can be conducted safely.

Personality characteristics and prognosis

Anxiety

ASPD is often linked with significant co-morbidities, especially substance misuse (Compton et al., 2005). Half of those with ASPD also have anxiety disorders (Goodwin & Hamilton, 2003), and a quarter experience depression (Lenzenweger et al., 2007). The presence of anxiety or depression can improve treatment outcomes, as patients are more likely to engage due to the distress caused by these conditions (Gabbard & Coyne, 1987). Anxiety may also indicate a capacity for healthier object relationships, which is necessary to form a therapeutic alliance with the therapist and is a prerequisite for the effectiveness of any therapeutic modality.

Attachment and object relations

Psychoanalytic and psychodynamic therapies rely on the therapeutic relationship between patient and therapist, with the unconscious dynamics of transference and countertransference serving as the core driver of therapeutic change. Patients lacking a capacity for attachment are less likely to form a meaningful relationship with the therapist in which these dynamics can be interpreted. Moreover, they may pose an increased risk to professionals, as empathy, which would normally inhibit aggression, is absent. The more severe the psychopathy, the more the patient is likely to interact with others based on power rather than affection (Meloy, 1988). This often includes attempts to control staff and fellow patients, reinforcing their grandiose self-image while defending against anxiety through control of professionals.

Psychological affects and defences

As described earlier, patients with ASPD struggle to experience mature emotions like affection, guilt, remorse, sympathy, and loss, which are crucial for psychoanalytic and psychodynamic therapies which rely on emotional engagement with the therapist. However, they may simulate such emotions for manipulation or secondary gain, which may be difficult for therapists to detect. Their use of primitive defence mechanisms such as projection, devaluation, denial, projective identification, omnipotence, and splitting may predispose transference experiences to be enacted rather than contained and interpreted. For example, the psychopathic patient may use projective identification by unconsciously projecting negative emotions such as envy, aggression, or fear, to the clinician, viewing them as a threat to be diminished, and attempt to control the clinician through intimidation.

Superego characteristics

The presence of any superego development, such as rationalising antisocial acts to gain approval, is a positive prognostic sign. Mild to moderately psychopathic patients may exhibit harsh self-attitudes, indicating internalised values. However, severely psychopathic patients often display sadistic behaviour towards others without justification or remorse. These individuals should not be considered for treatment due to the risk they pose to staff and other patients. Therapy is unlikely to benefit psychopathic patients with sadistic aggression, absence of remorse, very superior intelligence or mildly intellectual disability, lack of emotional attachments, and those who provoke unexpected fear in experienced clinicians (Meloy & Yakeley, 2010).

General treatment considerations

Regardless of the therapeutic intervention offered, the difficulties in individuals with ASPD in forming meaningful attachments, including with professionals, compromises their engagement in treatment. It is important to address motivation for and engagement in therapy, as well as establishing the boundaries of treatment.

Motivation for therapy

When assessing the patient, discrepancies may arise between the motivations of the referring party and the patient. The primary aim of professionals may be the reduction of the patient's risk to others, while the person concerned may only be seeking treatment to comply with conditions, such as gaining early release or contact with children. Though some may experience anxiety or depression, many individuals with ASPD reject the traditional sick role and do not view themselves as therapy patients, as this is associated with shame or vulnerability. It is therefore crucial to assess the individual's motivation for treatment and whether it aligns with that of the referrer.

Engagement in therapy

Those patients who may benefit from psychodynamic psychotherapy may require an extended initial period of engagement, stabilisation, and motivational work to foster a collaborative therapeutic alliance. Challenges such as missed sessions, aggression, crises, and substance abuse should be anticipated. Preparing patients with practical advice, psychoeducation, and treatment explanations may be necessary. To minimise drop-out and noncompliance, therapists may need to be more proactively involved than in non-forensic psychotherapeutic work, reminding patients of appointments, liaising with other professionals, and addressing issues like substance misuse, self-harm, housing, and chaotic lifestyles.

Boundaries

As many antisocial individuals view relationships through a lens of power and control, issues of dominance and hierarchy will affect any treatment. Their distrust or contempt for authority manifests in rebellion against rules and boundaries, and the ability of more psychopathic patients to charm and manipulate may lead professionals into boundary violations, including inappropriate social or sexual relationships. Many may have been involved in gangs or criminal subcultures with their own codes of conduct, which should be explored in therapy. Understanding these dynamics is crucial for effective treatment.

The ensuing case example illustrates some of these issues in the assessment of a patient with ASPD.

Luke, a 41-year-old white man, was referred to a specialist foren-sic psychotherapy service due to aggression, long-standing person-ality difficulties, depression, and a history of childhood trauma and abuse. Persecuted by feelings of rejection and ostracization by others triggered violent and suicidal thoughts and anxieties that he would act on. His mental state had deteriorated since stopping individual therapy one year ago and the break-up of a "relation-ship" with a woman he had become infatuated with at Alcoholics Anonymous (AA) 4 years previously. She initially reciprocated his attraction but quickly stopped contact and took out an injunc-tion against him, leaving him feeling hurt, rejected, and angry, and harbouring fantasies that he would stalk and attack her.

He expressed long-standing anger with both his parents – a violent and alcoholic father, now deceased, and a mother, still alive, who did not protect him from his father's abuse. He struggled academi-cally and was sent to a school for childhood behavioural problems. From age 13 he became involved in theft, stealing cars, and dealing drugs with other youths. He had convictions of violence towards women as well as men, often involving alcohol.

He admitted to many brief sexual encounters with women but no long-term relationships and described himself as jealous and possessive, hating women in general, especially his mother and the mother of his daughter. At age 22, he was convicted for actual bodily harm after hitting his then pregnant girlfriend, who he believed had been flirting with other men. He had never met his daughter, now age 18. A few years previously, he had assaulted his mother in a rage by hitting her and pull-ing her hair after he discovered she was seeing his daughter without his knowledge. He showed little remorse but also described a self-destructive streak in which he would end relationships to pre-empt rejection.

He had an extensive psychiatric history. He began drinking heavily in his teens, becoming alcoholic by his twenties. He had had multiple treatment attempts for the past 15 years through AA. After two inpatient admissions for overdoses in his early twenties, he attended low-fee therapy but left, insisting he deserved free treatment. At 30, a trauma clinic psychiatrist recommended a therapeutic community, which he refused, wanting treatment from her instead. Following an assault on his mother, he was referred to forensic services but not treated due to his ASPD diagnosis. He was also declined by an outpatient psychology service for aggression. Later, he joined the therapeutic community but was discharged after starting a sexual relationship with a patient. He then sustained four years of free therapy until it ended due to boundary issues. Referred to a personality disorder service via primary care, he was again rejected due to the risk he posed.

At the forensic psychotherapy service, he was assessed by a male therapist, who felt dismissed and controlled by his demand to have therapy with a woman and his refusal to be under the care of his local mental health service, who would provide co-working and additional psychiatric support if he were accepted for forensic psychotherapy.

In formulating his difficulties, we can postulate that his childhood experiences of abuse and neglect from parents who were unable to provide adequate nurturing and containment interfered in the normal process of attachment, resulting in poor affect regulation, impulsivity, and a limited capacity for mentalisation and intimate relationships with others. His internal world is dominated by primitive affects – shame, rage, contempt – and primitive defence mechanisms – denial, splitting, projection, idealisation – exemplified in his relationship with women, who are either idealised or denigrated. He uses both self-preservative and sadomasochistic violence to bolster an underlying sense of confusion and low self-esteem, and to defend against feelings of anger towards his parents, especially his mother. The presence of depression and primitive superego functioning in his punitive attitudes towards himself might indicate some positive prognosis in treatment, but his tendency to sabotage relationships and destroy good objects, including offers of help, manifested itself in his periods of individual psychotherapy in which it appears he was contained for some time before he violated their boundaries (his non-payment of fees and demand for social contact with the therapist). Moreover, although he could appear insightful and make links, it was unclear whether this was a product of intellectualisation and simulation rather than the internalisation of anything meaningful from either period of therapy.

In the transference, his aggressive demand for individual therapy with a female represents a wish for an exclusive relationship with the mother, which he defends against with anger and contempt towards the male assessing clinician, whose countertransference feelings of being scorned and humiliated reflect the projection of the patient's own unwanted feelings of rejection. Any attempt to separate by bringing in a third paternal figure (e.g. involving external agencies) is resisted and attacked. This dynamic is reflected in him not being accepted or discharged by mental health services, a repetition of his early experiences of care, leaving him feeling rebuffed and enraged, with increased risk of violence.

This chapter has used a psychoanalytically-informed conceptual framework to elucidate some of the general principles that should be tended to in the assessment and intervention for any patient with ASPD. The next chapter provides a critical appraisal of both historical and contemporary psychoanalytic and psychodynamic treatment modalities and techniques that have been developed for the disorder, with particular emphasis on the empirical evidence supporting their efficacy.

Chapter 7

Specific therapies for antisocial personality disorder

Treatment for ASPD: The empirical evidence

The early literature on treating antisocial patients with individual psychoanalytic therapy and group psychotherapy primarily relied on case reports, often excluding the most disturbed individuals (McGauley et al., 2007). Due to their dangerous behaviours such as violence and substance abuse, treatment in institutional settings was recommended to contain risks, but general psychiatric hospitals were often not suitable, as such patients tended to disrupt wards and manipulate staff (Gabbard, 2005).

This led to the development of specialised institutional settings for the treatment of antisocial and psychopathic patients and offenders. Here, the environmental setting, or milieu, becomes an essential therapeutic tool of the therapy, in which behaviour can be challenged and modified. The democratic therapeutic community (DTC) is a long-standing psychodynamic model of treatment which started in the UK over 50 years ago, having developed from interest in group treatments following the Second World War (Jones, 1952). In a DTC, all the patient members of the community take responsibility for both the care and containment of each other. Treatment is delivered mainly through large and small group sessions, where members challenge each other's behaviour based on community-developed rules. Peer support and collaborative problem-solving are key, with staff serving as facilitators rather than leading therapeutic change.

In the UK, early research on therapeutic community treatment focused on the Henderson Hospital, an NHS-funded residential

DOI: 10.4324/9781003559801-11

community. Therapeutic communities have also been implemented in prisons, notably HMP Grendon Underwood, which specialises in treating male prisoners with personality disorders. Other residential treatments tried for ASPD include token economy programmes, which reward good behaviour; and wilderness programmes, which promote responsibility and social skills through nature. However, although studies have shown improvements in symptomatology and personality change, there are no controlled outcome studies proving their effectiveness, and more psychopathic individuals may struggle to maintain pro-social behaviours once reintegrated into the community (Meloy & Yakeley, 2013).

In the 1990s, studies showed that therapeutic communities (TCs) led to poorer outcomes and higher drop-out rates for psychopaths, even increasing violent recidivism (Ogloff et al., 1990; Harris et al., 1994), reinforcing the belief that psychopathy was untreatable. Though later refuted (McGuire, 2022), this led to a shift from psychodynamic approaches to cognitive-behavioural and social skills programmes targeting behaviours like aggression and substance abuse (Yakeley & Meloy, 2012).

Political concern over public safety following high-profile homicides spurred the development of treatment programmes for offenders with severe personality disorders. In Canada, offender-focused treatment programmes emerged (Wong et al., 2007), while the UK established intensive units for individuals with "dangerous and severe personality disorder" (Department of Health & Home Office, 1999). This evolved into the Offender Personality Disorder (OPD) Pathway, a government-funded initiative providing psychologically informed services across health and criminal justice sectors to reduce reoffending and improve mental health (Joseph & Benefield, 2012). Rooted in relational and attachment theory, the OPD Pathway incorporates psychoanalytic principles, offering interventions like mentalisation-based treatment (MBT), therapeutic communities, and psychologically informed planned environments (PIPEs). Although many in the Pathway likely meet ASPD criteria, they are not routinely identified as such, except within the MBT trial (see below).

Only a small number of high-quality randomised controlled treatment trials have been conducted among people with ASPD

(Gibbon et al., 2010; 2020). However, a comparative evaluation of available studies has been hampered by different diagnostic criteria and conceptualisations of psychopathy versus ASPD, differences in defining and measuring outcome, small sample sizes, short follow up periods, focus on treating incarcerated patients rather than those in the community, and an emphasis on behavioural and symptomatic rather than structural personality change.

Individual psychodynamic psychotherapy

Despite the lack of empirical evidence for its efficacy, and the many therapeutic challenges and risks involved, committed and experienced psychoanalytic and psychodynamic clinicians continue to engage in psychodynamic psychotherapy with patients diagnosed with ASPD. They have also contributed to the ongoing research and refinement of therapeutic techniques tailored to this population, for whom traditional psychoanalytic methods are often unsuitable.

Only a minority of patients with a diagnosis of ASPD will benefit from psychodynamic psychotherapy. Providing sufficient expertise and support for the therapy is available, the normal threshold for offering psychodynamic therapy will need to be lowered, as patients with ASPD will not fulfil conventional suitability criteria such as psychological mindedness and ego strength. The assessment process aims to ascertain whether the patient's potential for curiosity in his internal world and ownership of his difficulties can be nurtured and developed. As described earlier, favourable selection criteria include low to moderate levels of psychopathy, presence of anxiety and/or depressive affect, a history of some capacity to form attachments with other people, the presence of higher-level or neurotic defences, and some evidence of superego functioning.

From the outset, therapeutic techniques should be adapted to meet the specific needs of the patient with ASPD, forming part of the spectrum of strategies employed to foster engagement. For example, therapists may need to intervene more actively or be flexible with the duration of sessions at the beginning of therapy, as patients who are particularly anxious or paranoid may find silences threatening or experience the standard session length as overwhelming. Patients are unlikely to be able to tolerate intensive therapy, so the frequency of therapy is usually no more than once weekly.

Therapeutic interventions should be carefully timed and calibrated in response to the patient's emotional state. A central task is to help the patient begin to access unconscious material without provoking overwhelming anxiety, aggression, or despair in either the patient or therapist. Early interpretations of unconscious conflict or fantasy should be avoided, as these often exceed the patient's limited capacity for symbolic thinking and internal representation. Instead, brief, straightforward observations about the patient's emotional state are typically more effective. This can involve the therapist naming the patient's concrete feelings and thoughts and gradually introducing metaphors to foster symbolic thinking. The therapist plays a key role in helping the patient link internal emotional states to outward behaviours, enabling the patient to begin recognising how acts of violence or substance misuse can serve as defences against more painful or distressing internal experiences.

For patients whose early caregivers were abusive or neglectful, the experience of being genuinely thought about by another person may feel both unfamiliar and threatening. A key therapeutic goal is to gradually create a mental space within the patient where differences, such as those between self and other, can be tolerated rather than feared. This process involves the slow internalisation of the therapist as a dependable, consistent, and empathic figure, who maintains clear boundaries, withholds judgment, and is open to multiple perspectives. Many individuals with ASPD have faced significant early disruptions in the processes of separation and individuation, with their minds and bodies treated as narcissistic extensions of their parents' minds and bodies rather than recognised as autonomous. Psychotherapy helps these patients begin to discover and inhabit transitional mental spaces, as described by Winnicott (1953), where playfulness, imagination, and exploratory relating can emerge and be safely experienced.

However, many of these patients are unlikely to tolerate a free-associative approach, and the therapeutic work may need to be more structured and directive than is typical in classical psychoanalytic therapy. Interpretations should concentrate more on the immediate, present-moment dynamics – the "here and now" – rather than attempting to reconstruct past experiences, although gaining an understanding of the childhood antecedents of their adult difficulties may also be therapeutic. While the therapist remains attuned to transference throughout the treatment, the process of directly interpreting it in the classical sense, by exploring how the patient's perception of the therapist is shaped by early relational patterns, may need to be deferred until the later stages of therapy. Patients with ASPD often communicate in a concrete and one-dimensional manner, making it difficult or even impossible for them to engage with the symbolic or "as-if" nature of transference. Instead, they tend to identify with the literal content of interpretations, rather than grasping their deeper symbolic meaning.

Moreover, for patients with a fragile sense of self who perceive the world as threatening and punitive, early interpretations of negative transference should be avoided. Such interpretations are likely to be experienced as critical or retaliatory, reinforcing the patient's belief that the world, and the therapist, are composed solely of hostile or malevolent figures.

Given the extent of psychological damage often present in these patients with ASPD, therapeutic goals should remain modest, aiming for small, gradual shifts in the patient's internal world. A key difficulty lies in the paradox that increased self-awareness often brings greater psychological distress. If insight emerges too rapidly, patients may become overwhelmed and regress into familiar pathological patterns. Therapy frequently involves cycles of progress followed by setbacks, including depressive withdrawal or impulsive behaviour, both defences against self-reflection. Gains made in one session may be dismissed or attacked in the next. These patterns reflect shifts between paranoid-schizoid and depressive positions, as described by Klein (1975 [1946]) and Bion (1962). Therapeutic progress involves helping the patient tolerate ambivalence and move towards the depressive position, where they can begin to acknowledge loss, tolerate conflicting emotions, and replace blame and grievance with guilt and concern.

At the same time, therapists must be cautious not to be misled by the apparent progress of psychopathic patients, who may consciously or unconsciously simulate emotional maturity to meet perceived expectations. Glasser (1996) described this as "simulation", a form of insincere compliance that may not be fully conscious. Cartwright (2002) highlights patients' "pseudo-digestive capacities", where they may briefly discuss their offence with apparent remorse, only to never revisit it, indicating superficial rather than genuine engagement. These dynamics can be subtle and difficult to detect, sometimes only sensed intuitively as something inauthentic or unsettling in the patient's presentation. Glasser (1996) warns that such simulations can distort the therapeutic process. This highlights the importance of monitoring countertransference, not only to better understand the patient's inner world but also to prevent the therapist from unconsciously colluding with the patient's defences or engaging in enactments.

Group analytic therapy

Whilst there has been some research and evidence into psycho-analytic or psychodynamic group work with offenders in secure hospitals, prison settings, and the community (Adshead, 2015; Maxwell-Scott, 2021), there have been no high-quality studies evaluating the efficacy of this treatment approach in antisocial personality disorder. Nevertheless, case studies and clinical experience suggest that group analytic therapy for many antisocial and psychopathic patients may be more effective than individual therapy (Meloy & Yakeley, 2013). Foulkes (1983 [1948]) was an early advocate for group analysis for individuals he described as socially "deviant", proposing that within a group patients could collectively form a norm from which they individually deviate. This highlights a striking paradox in the use of therapeutic groups for individuals with deviant or dangerous behaviours: rather than reinforcing antisocial tendencies, as might occur in prison or gang settings, participation in a structured therapeutic group, where individuals see their own struggles reflected in others, share experiences, and realise they are not alone in seeking autonomy and healthier relationships can help diminish such behaviours and foster meaningful psychological change (Schlapobersky, 1996).

For patients with underdeveloped mentalising abilities, group therapy may be more effective than individual treatment. The group can serve as both a container for the patient's projections and a collective auxiliary ego, helping to think and reflect on behalf of the individual. Over time, this process can support the gradual development of healthier ego functioning.

People with ASPD often prefer hierarchical relationships, and group dynamics can highlight their sensitivity to authority and related distortions in thinking. They also tend to over-control emotions within structured attachments, which can manifest as avoidance or ambivalence, behaviours that become visible in groups. Group therapy can help address their emotional deficit in experiencing social emotions like guilt, love, and fear that usually inhibit violence. Finally, if emotional recognition difficulties extend beyond fear and sadness, treatment should emphasise improving awareness of all emotions in oneself and others (Bateman, 2022). Additional therapeutic benefits of the group setting include the modelling of appropriate behaviours and interpersonal interactions, which patients can begin to internalise and adopt in their own relationships.

Antisocial patients with impaired reality testing are at risk of developing intense transference relationships in individual therapy, which may take on erotic or psychotic dimensions. These individuals often fare better in group therapy, where transference is spread across multiple group members, helping to diffuse the emotional intensity, which is one reason why violent impulses may be more effectively contained and explored within a group context (Welldon, 1996). Group therapy is also particularly well-suited for psychopathic individuals whose behaviour is marked by secrecy, manipulation, and deception, including those who have committed sexual offences. In a group of peers with similar tendencies, it becomes more difficult for the individual to maintain a false persona, as others are often able to recognise, challenge, and expose the subtle patterns of deception that shape the psychopath's interactions.

Empirically supported psychological therapies

More recently, specific evidence-based psychological therapies originally developed for borderline personality disorder have been adapted and show some promise in the treatment of antisocial behaviour. Though grounded in differing theoretical models, they share some overlapping techniques. From the cognitive-behavioural tradition, dialectical behaviour therapy (Linehan, 1993) and schema-focused therapy (Young et al., 2003) are the most prominent modalities but have not been trialled for ASPD. Transference-focused psychotherapy (TFP) and mentalisation-based treatment (MBT) are the most well-established therapies that have emerged from the psychoanalytic tradition. Over the past 20 years, adaptations of TFP have been trialled for forensic patients, including sexual offenders, in Austria and Germany (Fontao et al., 2006) but not specifically for patients with a diagnosis of ASPD. It is MBT that has accumulated the most convincing evidence to date as an effective psychological intervention for ASPD.

Mentalisation-based treatment

Mentalisation-based treatment (MBT) is a structured, time-limited, evidence-based psychological therapy that was originally developed in the 1990s to treat patients with borderline personality disorder in a partial day hospital setting. It is a psychodynamic therapy that incorporates relational and cognitive elements, and its theoretical frame of reference includes developmental psychology, attachment theory, and a theory about the mechanism of therapeutic action (Bateman & Fonagy, 2012). MBT is specifically focussed on increasing the capacity to mentalise.

MBT was initially shown to be effective in an RCT in patients with borderline personality disorder, where it diminished suicidal and self-injurious behaviours, significantly improved interpersonal functioning, and reduced the number of hospitalisations and use of medication compared to the control group (Bateman & Fonagy, 1999; 2001; 2009). MBT has subsequently been adapted for other disorders, including ASPD (Bateman & Fonagy, 2008; 2016). A recent large RCT (Fonagy et al., 2025) conducted within the OPD Pathway and involving 313 violent male offenders with ASPD found that those receiving 12 months of MBT-ASPD alongside probation had 50% lower aggression levels than those receiving probation alone. The MBT-ASPD group also showed a greater reduction in ASPD symptoms and committed 46% fewer offences over a three-year follow-up. This study offers the strongest evidence to date that a psychodynamic therapy can reduce aggression and criminal behaviour in ASPD.

Some of MBT's key strategies and interventions are elaborations of the modifications of technique of individual and group psychodynamic psychotherapy for antisocial patients described above. These include a focus on the patient's mind, not their behaviour; addressing current events and immediate states of mind rather past events or unconscious processes and fantasy; a stepwise intervention process starting with empathic validation of their experience, through clarification, affect elaboration, affect focus, and challenge; monitoring arousal levels; mentalising the transference and countertransference; and constantly monitoring the patient's mentalising capacity as well as maintaining or regaining the mentalising capacity of the therapist (Bateman & Fonagy, 2016). The therapist adopts a therapeutic stance of humility stemming from a sense of "not-knowing"; conveying authenticity, directness, respect, and courtesy, whilst avoiding opaquencss, hesitancy, and secrecy; and in which the patient's mental states and experiences are the object of joint attention and actively questioned, and where differences in perspectives are identified, legitimised, and accepted. This capacity of working together, of joint attention and shared intentionality (the ability to engage in shared, goal-directed activity), is known as "we-mode" or "we-ness" and is fundamental to healthy social interactions and prosocial behaviour but is lacking in individuals with ASPD, who struggle to maintain integrated and balanced mentalising (Bateman, 2022). The development of we-ness is supported by two group processes which are central to MBT-ASPD: agreeing on shared values and fostering relational mentalising to encourage compassion and sensitivity towards themselves and others.

MBT-ASPD addresses mentalising vulnerabilities in ASPD and is focussed on the following areas in relation to the dimensions of mentalising: 1. Understanding emotional cues: external mentalising and its link to internal states; 2. Recognition of emotions in others: other/affective mentalising; 3. Exploration of sensitivity to hierarchy and authority: self/cognitive; 4. Generation of an interpersonal process to understand subtleties of others' experience in relation to ones' own: self/other mentalising; 5. Explication of threats to loss of mentalising, for a teleological understanding of motivation: self/other mentalising and self/affective mentalising (Bateman et al., 2013).

The format of MBT-ASPD is a slow-open group with weekly sessions lasting 75 minutes, usually delivered by two therapists, and monthly individual sessions with one of the group therapists, and where patients are treated for 12 months. The first six to eight sessions function as an introductory and engagement phase (MBT-I), where the participants receive some psychoeducation regarding the concept of mentalisation, including discussions of the nature of emotions, facial expressions, and other nonverbal behaviours in order to stimulate an understanding of emotional cues, as well as how relationships can be defined by mutuality or hierarchy (Bateman et al., 2013). During these initial sessions, the group agrees on and defines a set of values; for example, respect, tolerance, mutuality, tolerance of different perspectives, and independence, which will inform the culture of the group and how it operates. These values are revisited and refined when new members start.

MBT-ASPD groups use several structured elements to support relational mentalising. Each session begins with a social check-in, where participants talk about their week – sharing experiences, voicing complaints, giving or receiving advice, and discussing significant events. This encourages connection and prosocial engagement. The clinician then summarises the previous session, focusing on relational dynamics within the group. After this, each participant is asked if there's anything they'd like to discuss with the group and whether there's someone specific they want to address. This process promotes interpersonal decision-making and emotional awareness. The session then moves into deeper exploration of participants' relationships, both within the group and in their daily lives, reinforcing the development of mentalising and social understanding (Bateman, 2022). Over time this leads to increasing affective understanding of self and others and the identification of relational patterns via increasing constructive interaction and decreasing destructive interaction (Bateman et al., 2019).

Patients with ASPD may become easily emotionally aroused or argumentative, losing any capacity to mentalise, often triggered by perceived slights from other patients or the therapists. It is important that the latter do not fall into joining non-mentalising discussions or arguing with the content of non-mentalising descriptions of others which may sound racist, misogynist, or denigratory in other ways. The therapists should try to track the non-mentalising process and get mentalising back on track, with techniques such as "stop and rewind" and "micro-slicing" of the non-mentalising speech or description (Bateman & Fonagy, 2016).

Moreover, patients with ASPD will often shape and experience the group as a hierarchal structure in which the therapists are in control, which they resent and resist. To avoid assuming such a position of authority and to counteract, the therapist should readily apologise for perceived errors and accept criticism to counteract the patient's expectations that the therapists hold all the power. This models the ability to accept mistakes and mis-understandings without losing mutual respect and compassion.

Finally, in order to foster self-other mentalising, the therapist may on occasion judiciously mentalise their countertransference experience to the patient, without inappropriate self-disclosure. This is not usually advocated in traditional psychoanalytic psy-chotherapy but is used in MBT-ASPD to stimulate the develop-ment of empathic empathy in patients by making them explicitly aware of the effects they have on others' minds, which is a key aspect of pro-social relationships.

The following clinical vignette from an MBT-ASPD group ses-sion illustrates some of the techniques which facilitate self-other affective mentalising.

This MBT group of six men with ASPD was facilitated by two therapists, a man and a woman. On this occasion, the male therapist was away, and the female therapist took the group session on her own. The group started with the men checking in about how they'd been in the last week. Leroy said he was feeling agitated as he'd been stopped and searched by a police-man and was convinced it was racist profiling as he was black. The other patients agreed that all police were racist and not to be trusted (psychic equivalence mode thinking). Tom, who was Spanish, started relating a story about how he was sometimes mistaken as being mixed race, and so he knows what it is like (this is also psychic equivalence – the assumption that he knows how Leroy feels). The others laughed and started talking about how you can't trust the authorities (the group had now entered pretend mode, talking about generalised issues in the external world and had lost touch with the heightened emotional state that Leroy had brought into the room).

The therapist recognised that the group were non-mentalising and that whilst this was part of their bonding and developing prosocial attitudes towards each other, she wanted to get mentalising back on track. She said that some strong opinions were being voiced about those in power in the external world, but perhaps we could come back to the work in the group. She reminded them that the previous week they had been discussing how they could misinterpret people's facial expressions and assume others were thinking or feeling something that might not be accurate. She asked what people wanted to talk about today.

Tony said he wanted to talk about an incident on the bus the day before which had made him angry. A large man sat down next to him, shoving his shoulder, and didn't apologise. Tony said he knew the man was baiting him as he had a nasty look on his face, and he could have sat in an empty seat behind him, so he asked the man what his problem was. The man asked him what his problem was, which made Tony "lose it" and swear at the man, which led to the bus driver stopping the bus and asking Tony to get off, leaving him feeling furious and humiliated.

Dennis said he was fed up hearing these stories from Tony. He said Tony was always getting into arguments with people on public transport, and he seemed to not be able to learn from the group, like misinterpreting people's facial expressions. Tony became visibly agitated and raising his voice told Dennis that he must think he was stupid. Dennis retorted that Tony shouldn't have started the argument with the man on the bus. Tony then stood up and said he was going to leave if he continued to be insulted by Dennis and that that was better than hitting him, which he felt like doing. Tony added that the therapist should tell Dennis that what he was saying was unacceptable.

At this point, the therapist intervened and asked Tony to sit down. She said she was wondering what state of mind Tony was in before he got on the bus. (Here the therapist is attempting to deescalate the situation and shift the focus temporarily by initiating an "MBT loop"– a brief diversion from the emotionally charged content that was disrupting Tony mentalising by encouraging him to reflect on his self-states before the bus incident rather than concentrating on the immediate tension in the session.) Tony admitted he was already irritable as he had just finished talking on the phone to his sister, who said she didn't want him to come to her daughter's party as she was afraid he'd pick an argument with her husband as he had done last time.

The therapist then asked what others thought about it (this is triangulation to create a space for different perspectives and lower the emotional tension). Gary said Tony was often paranoid, which they all were, and maybe the man just bumped into him by mistake and Tony didn't realise. Pete said he sympathised with Tony as he felt people should apologise, but maybe Tony shouldn't have kicked off.

The therapist, seeing that Tony appeared calmer, suggested that they rewind and think about what had just happened between Tony and Dennis, and asked Dennis why he had challenged Tony. Dennis said he recognised a pattern in Tony in how he was quick to become aggressive to others, and that perhaps he was similar but didn't like to admit it. Maybe he had been too confrontational with Tony too quickly, like Tony was with the man on the bus.

The therapist said she could see how quickly arguments could escalate and had felt a bit anxious herself when Tony had mentioned his urge to hit Dennis (the therapist is revealing her countertransference to facilitate Tony in being aware of the impact of his actions on others). Tony said she shouldn't have been anxious because he hadn't assaulted Dennis and also that he would never hit a woman (Tony demonstrates his lack of empathy with the therapist's affective state by offering a teleological explanation – that only a physical change is taken as proof that a mental state is real.). The therapist gently said that perhaps Tony didn't realise how he could appear threatening to others, but she was also aware that Tony wanted her to step in at that point, and she was curious to know what was in his mind. (Here the therapist is mentalising his relationship

*with her to move Tony out of psychic equivalence into menta-
lising. She does not interpret the transference or make links to
patterns of relationships external to the therapy setting or in
childhood as one would in psychoanalytic psychotherapy to
enhance insight; for example, suggesting that he might feel
persecuted by her like his sister, or that he felt unsupported by
the male therapist not being there, linked to his absent father in
childhood.) Tony said he'd thought she couldn't understand his
life being middle class and a woman, but perhaps he was being
paranoid and apologised for scaring her. Leroy said he admired
Tony for apologising, which was perhaps difficult for them all
to do especially when they feel disrespected.*

Future directions

MBT holds promise as an effective therapy for ASPD in a forensic
population, although more studies are needed in broader populations, such as those that commit intimate partner violence, and more
accessible community services for ASPD within both criminal justice
and health systems need to be developed. In the UK, TCs in secure
settings offering a psychodynamic framework within which a range
of psychological interventions are delivered continue to be developed
and evaluated, marking a resurgence of interest in psychodynamic
approaches to the treatment of offenders with personality disorders,
most commonly ASPD.

Part 4

Special populations

Chapter 8

The antisocial woman

Female offenders

ASPD and psychopathy are conditions more frequently associated with men. Women who are antisocial, kill their partners, neglect or abuse their children, or defraud and con others attract media attention, moral panic, and vicarious fascination for affronting conventional notions of femininity and maternal care, impeding serious exploration divorced from sensationalisation. Moreover, female violence and offending is often judged more harshly than male antisocial behaviours, and women are either overly punished for transgressing feminine norms or under-recognised as capable of serious harm.

It was not until the feminist movement of the 1970s and 1980s that there was any serious and sustained interest in female offenders (Yakeley, 2010). Feminist criminologists challenged earlier biological theories of female violence, instead emphasising social, economic, and structural factors in female offending, arguing that female violence could not be understood outside of patriarchal structures. Violence by women was seen as reactive, linked to histories of abuse, poverty, or marginalisation. The focus of interest shifted from street crime to domestic violence, a hidden and shameful sphere. Women were now understood as being victims, not perpetrators, of physical and sexual abuse, typically by male partners.

The psychiatrist and group analyst Estela Welldon's book *Mother, Madonna, Whore* (1988) sparked controversy and public outrage by suggesting mothers could abuse their children. Her

DOI: 10.4324/9781003559801-13

work prompted psychoanalysis and the nascent discipline of forensic psychotherapy to explore the origins and psychodynamics of female violence, proposing that some women may unconsciously use their bodies, partners, or children to express needs in violent or perverse ways. Before examining the work of Welldon and others in this area, it is helpful to review some of the empirical findings in relation to gender differences in ASPD and psychopathy.

ASPD in women: Empirical findings

Many of the first studies on ASPD were in male samples only, and scientific interest in antisocial behaviour in women dates mostly from the 1990s. More recent epidemiological studies show that ASPD presents in a ratio 3:1 of males to females regardless of age or ethnicity (Alegria et al., 2013), with a prevalence in the general population of 0.2–1% in women compared to 2–6% in men. As with ASPD in men, the prevalence of ASPD is significantly raised in women in prison settings, with rates of 47% of incarcerated male offenders and 21% of female offenders meeting diagnostic criteria for ASPD (Fazel & Danesh, 2002). ASPD may also be underdiagnosed in women due to gender stereotyping, as well as DSM criteria that emphasise traits like irritability and disregard for safety, behaviours more common in males, potentially leading to diagnostic bias against recognising ASPD in females (Özel et al., 2025).

There is now a multitude of studies which show the presentation of ASPD, associated aetiological factors, and developmental trajectory differ significantly between men and women. Girls with conduct disorder are less likely to be physically aggressive than boys with the disorder but are more likely to truant from school and run away from home. Girls also tend to be more anxious but have higher levels of cognitive and affective empathy. In adults, behavioural differences between men and women with ASPD include females being more prone to desert or hit their spouse, and less likely to engage in violent or illegal behaviours such as arson, damage to property, assault, harming animals, or using weapons. In contrast to their male counterparts, their violence tends to be directed towards those closest to them, their partners or children, rather than strangers. Women are also more likely to be deceitful and impulsive, and less frequently aggressive, irritable, or reckless than men with ASPD. Additionally, women show greater perceived stress and decreased well-being, social and emotional functioning, and self-harming behaviours (Verona & Vitale, 2006). Moreover, women with ASPD report significantly higher rates of childhood emotional neglect, sexual abuse, parental mental illness or substance use disorder, and adverse events during adulthood compared to men with ASPD (Alegria et al., 2013).

Violence against the body

Women are more likely than men to internalise their aggression towards themselves and their bodies. Self-harm through cutting is one clear example, but disorders like anorexia nervosa and bulimia, or somatisation, may also be seen as internalised violence against the female body. Welldon challenged both the traditional psychoanalytic view and the feminist assumption that women are only victims, not perpetrators, of violence. She argued that women can be aggressive and violent, often in subtle or perverse ways, and that this violence may be directed not only at themselves but also at their children, questioning a deeply held societal belief that mothers are incapable of harming their offspring (Welldon, 1988).

All children must navigate the complex task of separating from their primary maternal figure to become independent. This process relies on the child's healthy aggressive impulses being tolerated by a "good-enough" mother (Winnicott, 1953). When a mother cannot tolerate her child's self-assertion and responds with rejection, retaliation, or withdrawal, the child becomes overwhelmed by unprocessed aggression, both their own and the mother's. To cope, the child may evacuate these feelings into others or turn them inwards. For girls, separation is more complex, as they share a similar body with their mother. Welldon suggests that girls, not being their mother's true sexual object, receive less investment and thus depend more heavily on her. If the mother impedes separation, the girl's identifications and internal objects remain confused and undifferentiated from the internal maternal object, making her more vulnerable to internalised aggression. In this context, self-harm can be understood as a symbolic attack on the internalised mother's body in an attempt to gain separation.

For violent women, including those with ASPD, who have experienced actual maternal abuse or neglect, the task becomes much harder. Consciously, they may idealise their abusive or neglectful mothers to preserve attachment and ensure psychological survival. However, this defends against a punitive and humiliating internalised image of the mother, and unconsciously the little girl identifies with the rejected, shamed aspects, resulting in conscious guilt and self-loathing. When separation from the mother fails, the girl's inner world fuses with this destructive maternal image. This may resurface in adolescence, triggered by biological changes, leading to internalising behaviours such as self-harm or disordered eating but also the externalisation of aggression in an effort to cope with the emerging conflict and separation from the maternal object. This aggression is more likely to be directed at the woman's children or partner.

Perverse motherhood

Maria's mother was frequently unwell throughout her childhood, suffering from unexplained stomach pains, headaches, and spells of breathlessness. During these episodes, she took to her bed and issued orders to her children, especially Maria, the eldest, who was expected to care for the household. Any defiance from Maria was met with emotional outbursts or threats of collapse. Maria's father remained distant, either working or drinking alone, and did not intervene. Maria started cutting herself as a teenager and developed vague physical complaints, nausea, dizziness, and abdominal pain, with no medical cause. She also became disruptive at school, initiating arguments and physical fights with other children.

At 16, Maria left home to live with an older boyfriend and soon became pregnant. The relationship was unstable, marked by frequent arguments and separations. When her infant son was brought to hospital with a fractured arm, Maria claimed he had rolled off the sofa. Further scans revealed multiple older fractures. Maria appeared tearful but vague, saying she was exhausted and may have dropped him. While being questioned, she began vomiting and complained of dizziness, though no physical cause was found. During a home visit, social workers found the flat dirty and disordered. Maria said she had been "too ill" to keep up with chores.

At first, Maria blamed her ex-partner for the injuries but later admitted he had left months before. She said she sometimes "blacked out" when the baby cried and wasn't sure what happened. Professionals noted emotional lability, inconsistent accounts, and a tendency to present herself as the victim. She often arrived at meetings with sudden physical complaints – chest pain, faintness – that resolved once attention shifted to her child.

Welldon (1988) proposed that some mothers choose motherhood for unconsciously perverse reasons, using their babies to fulfil unconscious needs and express unresolved internal conflicts, often in disturbing or violent ways. On a conscious level, a woman might hope to heal from her own abusive maternal experiences by becoming a mother herself. However, on an unconscious level, the child may come to symbolise a form of victorious revenge against her own mother. Through motherhood, the woman assumes a position of power and control over the child, mirroring the dominance once exerted over her by her own mother. In many cases, these women lack internalised good objects, leading to feelings of inner emptiness. As a result, pregnancy may unconsciously serve to feel psychologically filled or nourished.

When these women become mothers, they often struggle to perceive their children as separate, autonomous individuals, but instead relate to them as narcissistic extensions of themselves. The baby becomes a vessel for the mother's unresolved emotional needs, cravings for affection and nurturing, as well as a repository for her unresolved fear and aggression originally directed towards her own mother. This latent hostility often surfaces when the child begins to assert independence, disrupting the mother's illusion of a seamless, merged identity with her child. Such tensions typically emerge during critical developmental milestones involving separation, such as birth, weaning, taking first steps, and starting school.

These perceived threats of separation trigger unresolved separation anxieties rooted in the woman's internalised experiences of her own mother. This leads to aggressive responses in the woman, which in their more passive form may result in neglect of their child, but in other instances intense aggression may arise that cannot be contained and becomes enacted as actual violence towards her child. The forensic psychotherapist Anna Motz (2008) powerfully illustrates how the baby can become the receptacle of the mother's violent impulses, drawing from DeMause's (1990) concept of children as "poison containers". In this framework, infants are unconsciously used by their mothers as vessels for disowned and toxic emotional states.

Intimate Partner Violence (IPV)

Intimate Partner Violence (IPV) research has long been influenced by feminist theory, which attributes IPV to sexism and male power dynamics, viewing women's violence as defensive or socially conditioned. However, recent studies challenge this view, showing that women can perpetrate IPV at similar rates to men. These findings suggest that IPV motivations in both men and women often include retaliation, emotional expression, or self-defence, rather than a simple desire for control (Cannon et al., 2016). Women with ASPD are at higher risk of being both victims and perpetrators of IPV, which includes involvement in relationships characterised by mutual or bidirectional violence (Yakeley, 2022).

A psychoanalytic approach may shed further light on why abused women stay within IPV relationships, looking at the unconscious dynamics between victim and perpetrator that can sustain abusive relationships, without implying that they choose or deserve the abuse. Motz (2008) suggests the victim-victimiser bond may unconsciously meet psychological needs for both partners. Acknowledging the victim's unconscious participation is not to blame her but to move beyond seeing her as a passive victim with little agency.

The defence mechanisms of projection and projective identification help elucidate the unconscious dynamics in abusive relationships. The abusive man may project his feelings of inadequacy into his female partner, attacking her as an unconscious hated and denigrated version of himself. Less obvious, but equally significant, is the abused woman's unconscious role in accepting this projection. As explored above, women with histories of childhood abuse or neglect may have already internalised an identity as damaged, shaped by early exposure to parental violence and victimised mothers. Feelings of anger and aggression towards the abusive parents are associated with intense guilt and so are split off and directed against themselves, to preserve the parent as a good object. In adulthood, enduring abuse may unconsciously serve to manage this guilt and re-create familiar dynamics. Both partners are influenced by unresolved early object relationships: the man may unconsciously perceive his partner as an overpowering maternal figure, with violence becoming his way of asserting separateness. The woman, in turn, may unconsciously find a sense of power in being needed by a dependent and violent partner. Thus, both participants play complementary roles in a shared unconscious script rooted in past trauma and early attachment patterns, perpetuating the cycle of abuse while remaining largely unaware of their mutual psychological investment in it.

Such relationships can be viewed as containing sadomasochistic elements, with both partners dependent on the other, and both assuming at times unconscious sadistic and masochistic positions. As discussed in previous chapters, one of the hallmarks of sado-masochistic violence is that the object is preserved and not destroyed – within these couples, both partners unconsciously ensure that neither is destroyed nor abandoned. These relationships are often characterised by cycles in which the man is violent and the woman threatens to leave, followed by the man begging for her forgiveness and the woman deciding to give him another chance. The woman may unconsciously identify with both an abandoning object in her threats to leave but also with an abandoned child, represented in the present in her partner but based on her own experiences as a child, and she unconsciously wishes to protect her partner from the pain of being abandoned. Her internal oscillation between these two positions constitutes a central unconscious conflict that impedes her ability to separate from her partner. The relationship between battered wife and battering husband is one in which all the violence is overtly located in the man. However, this conceals unconscious dynamics in which both partners are locked in a sadomasochistic prison from which neither can escape. The woman's aggression may only become evident when she becomes violent herself and in rare cases kills her partner.

This exposes the false dichotomy that exists between viewing female offenders as either victims in which their antisocial behaviour has developed as a survival strategy against childhood trauma, or as the perpetrators of heinous crimes due to innate psychopathy, depicted as evil or "angels of death". As with ASPD, women with psychopathy report high levels of adverse childhood experiences and disruptions of attachment, and although personality traits such as lack of empathy may be due to having to dissociate from their emotions to cope with childhood abuse, or exploitation of others may be a tactic developed to ensure their emotional needs are met, this does not mean that the severity of their aggression and sadism should be overlooked and give rise to false therapeutic optimism and perpetuation of the belief that only men are true psychopaths.

Psychopathy in women: Empirical findings

As with ASPD, female psychopathy has been less well studied than psychopathy in men. It is less common than in males, with a reported prevalence on only 1.6% of UK female prisoners compared to 7.7% in males (Coid et al., 2009). However, bias in the assessment of psychopathy according to social norms may lead to underdiagnosis of psychopathy in women. For example, financial dependence on others may be viewed as acceptable behaviour in women but as parasitic behaviour in men.

Significant differences with regard to the expression of psychopathy between male and female psychopaths have been found in several key areas (Rogstad & Rogers, 2008). Female psychopaths are more likely to commit theft or fraud rather than violent crimes, which are more common in male psychopaths. Aggression is also expressed differently between the sexes. For women, this tends to be verbal, whereas men show more physical violence. For those female psychopaths who are violent, this is more likely to be more affective than predatory (Cunliffe et al., 2013; Meloy, 2006), and, like women with ASPD, the target of their violence is more frequently against people closest to them – i.e., their partners, children, and associates, rather than strangers (Greenfeld & Snell, 1999). Female psychopaths also tend to have higher levels of emotional instability and suicidality compared to male psychopathic offenders.

In their interpersonal relationships, female psychopaths show more interest and connection, and are more likely to seek approval from others, in contrast to the arrogance, detachment, callousness, and remorselessness exhibited by men with psychopathy (Cunliffe et al., 2013; Gacono & Meloy, 1994; Hare, 2003). Women are also more likely to flirt while men are more likely to run scams and commit fraud (Forouzan & Cooke, 2005). These behaviours may have different underlying motivations – in women promiscuous behaviour may reflect a wish to exploit their partners to gain financial benefits, or covertly influence their social networks, in contrast to men, who may be driven by sensation-seeking or a desire for sexual activity. Similarly, drug use in men may be linked to a pursuit for excitement driven by peer pressure, whereas in women, drug abuse may be more socially embedded and function as a coping strategy (Bloom et al., 2005).

Female psychopathy as malignant hysteria

Based on findings from using the Rorschach test in women with psychopathy (Cunliffe et al., 2013; Gacono & Meloy, 1994), Meloy and colleagues offer a psychoanalytic conceptualisation of female psychopathy as a form of "malignant hysteria", a more extreme version of hysterical or histrionic personality disorder, characterised by superficiality, egocentricity, vanity, dependence, manipulativeness, dramatic behaviour, and disturbed interpersonal relationships. This malignant hysterical personality style of the female psychopath differs from the malignant narcissism that characterises male psychopathy.

Compared to their male counterparts, on the Rorschach test, female psychopaths differ in exhibiting a negative self-image, emotional dysphoria, increased need for approval and attention, seductive or dramatic behaviour, and poor interpersonal relatedness. This suggests that, in contrast to the male psychopath, there is an absence of a grandiose self-structure, and instead, the female psychopath desires attention and acceptance from others to mediate the effects of chronic dissatisfaction and self-criticism. However, their reliance on others fails to regulate self-esteem and mood, resulting in dysphoric affect and negative oppositional feelings. Compared with non-psychopathic ASPD females, women with ASPD and psychopathy show diminished psychological resources, reduced stress tolerance, chronic self-criticism/negative sense of self, pathological self-focus in the absence of grandiosity, anger, interpersonal dependency, limited capacity for self-reflection and understanding the motives of others, lack of empathy, and poor reality testing.

Further Rorschach studies indicate that the psychodynamics of the female psychopathic personality is, like the male, organised at Kernberg's borderline level of functioning as evidenced by her reliance on the defence mechanisms of repression, isolation, devaluation, dissociation, and projection. However, in contrast to men with psychopathy, somatic complaints and significant dependency needs are common, which is consistent with a hysterical configuration (Smith et al., 2014). Moreover, female psychopaths appear to be strongly identified with a victim stance, suggesting a tendency to try to elicit sympathy from others as means of gaining attention, acceptance, and approval. They also demonstrate more sadomasochistic responses, which, alongside a compromised sense of self, may indicate that they derive satisfaction from harming others to fulfil unmet emotional needs or to bolster their diminished self-esteem.

Female psychopaths therefore lack the narcissistic grandiose self-structure of male psychopaths which acts to ward off external and internal threats to self-esteem but instead requires others to shore up their self-image. Unlike the male psychopath who basks in his self-image, the psychopathic woman needs others for mirroring and experiences disappointment and rejection when she is unable to attract others' attention and approval (Gacono & Smith, 2021). Because they do not exhibit the overtly dominant behaviour of the male psychopath, their presentation may be more subtle, and they are more able to charm and manipulate others, including professionals, into seeing them as victims and so they miss their psychopathy. Their need for affiliation and recognition by others may be misinterpreted as a genuine connection with others rather than a shallow, self-serving contact aimed at eliciting attention. Moreover, the female psychopath's dysphoric affect may be erroneously diagnosed as depression rather than a manifestation of character disturbance.

Treatment considerations

Compared to men, research into the causes, trajectory, and treatment of ASPD and psychopathy in women has been neglected, with a concomitant lack of available treatment interventions and services. Such women often present with complex psychopathology and needs, which include those of their children and families, necessitating the involvement of many different services within the health and criminal justice systems, social services, education, and victim support. Seeking help may be particularly shameful and dangerous for women whose offences have involved their children or partners, where they may be ostracised by or at risk of violent retaliation from their families or communities.

Such emotional responses may be reflected in professionals offering support and treatment, who may be unconsciously affected by complex countertransference reactions, ranging from sympathy and compassion to moral outrage and disgust at the idea that women could commit heinous crimes of child abuse or the murder of their partners. The patient's psychopathology, modes of offending, and internal object relationships will surface within the transference dynamics of the therapeutic relationship, in which oscillations between power and submission, deception and collusion, sadism and masochism, seduction and rejection, become manifest and reflect the tensions in integrating the identifications of perpetrator and victim within the minds of both the patient and professionals. Supervision and reflective spaces for clinicians and services treating and managing women with ASPD are important to disentangle and understand the interplay between the patients' projections and the team's defences and process emotional responses, to prevent enactments and reduce risk.

Psychodynamic treatment provision is to date limited for this patient cohort. Women with ASPD who have some capacity for reflection and insight may benefit from individual psychodynamic therapy if available. The development of MBT services for antisocial women is in its infancy but shows promise as an effective treatment. Treating women who have neglected or abused their children raises additional complexities, including liaising with social services, and managing loss and grief where children have been removed from their care. Clinicians must also manage the patient's risk to themselves in self-harm and suicide attempts, as well as their risk to others, and be proficient in employing effective therapeutic techniques aimed at reducing these behaviours by promoting emotional stability and impulse control.

Female offenders often find it more difficult to cope in forensic psychiatric facilities and criminal justice settings than men (Loucks, 1995), and single sex services, whether these are women-only secure units, female prisons, or MBT groups exclusive to women are required, not only because they have different psychological needs to men but also because they may feel threatened by men due to their histories of abuse by fathers, stepfathers, or male partners.

Finally, therapeutic expectations may need to be modified, particularly with women who are more psychopathic, where the prognosis is limited due to the difficulties in changing personality traits such as callousness and lack of empathy, deceitfulness, manipulativeness, and sadism, which bestow a sense of control and gratification in their relationships and are therefore harder to relinquish. Again, although their experiences of victimhood may be more apparent than male psychopaths, they may be just as treatment resistant, and rehabilitative efforts may need to be limited to risk management and behavioural control.

Chapter 9

The antisocial sex offender

Empirical findings

Personality disorder is common in sexual offenders, with ASPD and borderline personality disorder being the most frequent. Studies have shown that up to half of sexual offenders may have a diagnosis of ASPD. A diagnosis of ASPD also increases the risk of sexual, violent, and general recidivism in sexual offenders (Hanson & Morton-Bourgon, 2005). There is also some evidence that the type of personality disorder differs according to the sexual offence committed, with ASPD being more likely in offenders who commit rape rather than child molesters (Aromäki et al., 2002; Francia et al., 2010). However, there is a lack of studies reporting the incidence and types of sexual offending in ASPD populations, including the rates of paraphilic disorders, for example paedophilia, exhibitionism, sadism, or fetishism. Although the presence of paraphilic disorders increases the risk of offending in sexual offenders (Oronowicz-Jaśkowiak et al., 2024), the current diagnostic classification systems have limited research into this area. DSM-5 and ICD-11 have resisted specifying rape as a paraphilic disorder; moreover, not all offenders who molest children have paedophilic disorder. There is more research regarding the relationship between psychopathy, rather than ASPD, and paraphilic disorders, in particular sadistic paraphilic disorder, with studies showing that sexual offenders with higher psychopathy scores were more likely to have a sadistic paraphilia than those with moderate or low psychopathy scores (Papagathonikou & Marono, 2025;

DOI: 10.4324/9781003559801-14

Woodworth et al., 2013). These distinctions are important from a psychoanalytic perspective, where the perverse characteristics of sexual offending may be understood as the sexualisation of underlying anxieties in relation to intimacy and aggression, and the symptoms of paraphilic disorders may be conceptualised as the manifestations of unconscious processes related to personality pathology (Yakeley et al., 2025).

The recognition that sexual offending is multiply determined has led to several contemporary multifactorial theories of sexual offending which incorporate psychological, biological, cultural, and situational factors (e.g. Beech & Ward, 2004; Marshall & Marshall, 2000). However, such models neglect unconscious factors, including the role of sexualisation as a defence against unconscious anxiety and aggression.

As with the development of ASPD, the role of adverse childhood experiences (ACE) and attachment difficulties in the aetiology of sexual offending in adulthood has gained increasing recognition. Experiencing sexual abuse as a child is one of the most severe examples of an ACE and has a disproportionate aetiological effect on adult sexual offending and is also a significant factor associated with a diagnosis of ASPD (Marshall, 2022).

The erotic form of hatred

Psychoanalytic theories on sexual deviancy or perversion have utility in understanding the sexual fantasies and behaviours of the antisocial person. Freud's earliest writings on perversion conceptualised polymorphous perversion as infantile sexual impulses that had evaded repression (Freud, 1905). However, in his paper *Fetishism* (Freud, 1927), his focus shifted to viewing perverse behaviours and fantasies as psychological defences against castration anxiety. The idea of perversion as a defence was taken up by later psychoanalysts, who proposed that it not only shields the individual from castration threats but also from more primitive, pre-Oedipal anxieties and hostile feelings directed towards the maternal object.

The psychoanalyst Robert Stoller (1975) relocated the origins of perversion to the infant's early relationship with the mother. He defined perversion as "the erotic form of hatred", where underlying hostility serves as the primary motivation, masked by overt sexualisation expressed through fantasies and behaviours. This sexualisation reflects an unconscious fantasy of vengeful triumph over early trauma rooted in the pre-Oedipal attachment to the mother, whose perceived omnipotence impedes the infant's ability to separate and develop an autonomous self. In this framework, perversion becomes a means of achieving gratification through hostility, acting as a defence against deep-seated anxieties and trauma. These early wounds may not result from overt abuse, but rather from the mother's over-gratifying, narcissistic presence, which creates a world the infant cannot escape. As a result, the adult compulsively reenacts this early conflict, endlessly seeking the mother's exclusive attention – only to degrade and defile it in an aggressive bid to separate and "dis-identify" (Stoller, 1974) from an unconscious fantasy of an all-consuming maternal figure.

The core complex

This unbearable battle for the child around separation and individuation from the mother is crystallised in Glasser's concept of the "core complex" (Glasser, 1996), which builds on his typology of aggression as described in Chapter 4. The core complex is a specific constellation of interconnected feelings, thoughts, and attitudes, representing a very early conflict between the wish to be close to the mother and the fear of being overwhelmed by her. At the heart of the complex is a profound and enduring longing for deep emotional closeness – an intense desire to merge with another person, to experience a "state of oneness" or "blissful union". While such desires are common to everyone, in individuals who have experienced an early pathologically narcissistic relationship with the mother, these longings persist in a primitive and undeveloped form, remaining unmodified by later stages of psychological growth. Merging is no longer experienced as a temporary or fulfilling connection but is instead feared as a permanent loss of self – a total dissolution of one's separate identity from the other, evoking a deep fear of annihilation. To protect against this overwhelming anxiety, the individual withdraws from intimacy, maintaining a "safe distance" from others. However, this retreat leads to feelings of emotional isolation, abandonment, and diminished self-worth. These painful emotions then reignite the longing for connection, trapping the individual in a cyclical pattern of approach and withdrawal, the defining dynamic of the core complex.

Aggression plays a central role in the core complex. The ego's fear of annihilation – the terror of losing a distinct, separate existence – triggers an intense aggressive response. To protect the self, the object – the mother at this early stage of development – must be psychically attacked or destroyed. However, doing so also threatens the loss of the nurturing aspects of the mother: her love, security, and warmth. Faced with this dilemma, the infant is left with two options – either to withdraw into a narcissistic state or to deploy aggression to defend the self against the overwhelming, engulfing mother. This, Glasser proposes, is the origin of self-preservative aggression and violence.

However, expressing this aggression would leave the child at risk of total abandonment, which pushes the child to withdraw into a narcissistic state. This space provides temporary sanctuary but soon becomes contaminated with feelings of isolation and abandonment, giving rise to longings to be close to the maternal object once again. Glasser proposes that the child's solution is to sexualise his aggression and hostility towards the feared but needed maternal object to escape from the terrifying vicious circle of the core complex. Although the mother is now made to suffer and her suffering becomes a source of pleasure, the relationship with her is preserved. The object – originally the mother – no longer needs to be destroyed completely but remains alive to be dominated and controlled. Via the process of sexualisation, self-preservative aggression is converted to sadomasochistic aggression, which may be enacted in sadomasochistic violence.

The contributions of Stoller and Glasser offer significant insights into the nature of perversion. Rather than expressing mature sexuality, the fantasies and behaviours of the perverse individual serve as a means of using sexualisation to defend against deeply rooted, early anxieties in relationships. While Freud emphasised castration anxiety as the central driver of perverse behaviour, this perspective highlights more fundamental fears, such as those related to separation, abandonment, and helplessness, as primary motivating forces.

The facts of life

The psychoanalysts Roger Money-Kyrle (1971) and Janine Chasseguet-Smirgel (1984) extended the concept of sexualisation as a defence against these early pre-Oedipal anxieties to one in which sexualisation acts as a more global attack on reality itself, the denial and disavowal of sexual and generational difference. Money-Kyrle identifies three fundamental truths of human existence, which he calls the "facts of life" (Money-Kyrle, 1971). The first fact of life involves the infant's realisation of dependence on an external source for nourishment, confronting the fantasy of self-sufficiency and requiring an ability to tolerate both dependence and separation. The second concerns the recognition of generational and sexual difference: the awareness that the mother is a separate individual capable of forming a creative, intimate union with another – typically the father – to conceive a child, a relationship from which the child is necessarily excluded. The third truth involves coming to terms with the passage of time and the reality of mortality: the understanding that we age, are not all-powerful, and must learn to face loss and engage in the process of mourning.

Perverse sexuality, therefore, involves an attack on truth and the pursuit of pathological solutions aimed at denying these fundamental facts of life. For example, the paedophile erases generational boundaries by choosing a child as a sexual partner, thereby rejecting the reality of developmental difference. Similarly, those who engage in sadomasochistic sexual acts that centre on the pursuit of pain for sexual pleasure deny the creative and life-giving potential of sexual intercourse, instead transforming it into something destructive. Chasseguet-Smirgel (1984) characterised the perverse psyche as inhabiting an "anal-sadistic universe", where distinctions between generations and genders are denied. She saw perversions as omnipotent, magical attempts to avoid the traumatic recognition of sexual and generational differences – efforts to construct a reality in which these fundamental distinctions are erased. Within this distorted world, the penis, faeces, and child are seen as equivalent and interchangeable, reflecting a form of perverse "pseudocreativity" that substitutes illusion for genuine creative capacity.

At the age of 23, Mr C received a life sentence for murder. Although there was no overt history of parental abuse, little affection or emotion was expressed in the family. Mother was strict and prudish, and father went along with his wife's decisions regarding the discipline and upbringing of the children. Mr C described himself as a "bad" child from birth, "breaking all the boundaries" by shoplifting from the age of five, playing truant from school, and becoming involved in increasingly delinquent activities such as stealing cars and breaking into people's houses as a teenager. At the age of 11, Mr C started to engage in sexual activity with his younger sister, during which he would coerce her into what he described as "putting willies together". When he was 13, Mr C's sexual preoccupation with his sisters was replaced after he saw his mother naked in the shower. Thereafter, his mind was filled with sexual fantasies about his mother. He started to steal his mother's underwear and could only achieve orgasm on masturbation whilst dressed in his mother's bra and panties. At school, Mr C was bullied for a stammer and became a bully himself. From the age of 14 he started to abuse drugs and alcohol, and by the time he was 16 he was visiting prostitutes on a regular basis. These prostitutes were older women who reminded him of his mother. Prior to his index offence, Mr C had no convictions for violence, and by his own account did not consider himself to be a violent person.

On the night of the murder, Mr C had visited a prostitute but had failed to ejaculate due to alcohol inebriation. Discovering he had no money for a taxi, he decided to mug a passer-by for their wallet. He accosted a man and led him into a blind alley. The man, however, appeared to have thought that Mr C wanted sex and dropped his trousers. Mr C, fearing sexual assault, attacked him with a piece of wood lying on the ground. He fled the scene but returned five minutes later with the conscious decision to "finish him off so that he could not tell". He attacked him again so that the man sustained severe head inju-ries and died. Post-mortem examination of the body revealed that he had also been attacked by Mr C in his groin.

Although the psychodynamics of such a complex case are spec-ulative, it is clear in Mr C's perverse behaviour as a child and ado-lescent how sexual and generational boundaries are erased. His belief that his sister had the same anatomy as himself – they both possessed "willies" – defends against castration anxieties, and his desire to have his mother as his sexual partner denies the fact that she is of a separate generation and in a couple with his father. It is likely that Mr C's aggression towards his overbearing and controlling mother was sexualised at an early age in the perverse behaviour of cross-dressing in his mother's underwear. His aggression was more overt in his early boundary breaking – stealing and truancy – which was perhaps an unconscious attempt to gain the attention of his emotionally absent parents. The index offence can be understood as an enactment of his rage towards both his parents – his unobtainable mother and his ineffectual father. His initial violent attack on the man appears to be self-preservative violence, reacting in self-defence to the fear that he is being sexually assaulted. This fear taps into his own rejection of the passive homosexual position that he has unconsciously adopted in relation to his father, resulting from an Oedipal failure to identify with his father and separate from his mother. At the same time, Mr C feels rejected and humiliated by his sexual encounter with the prostitute, evidence that he cannot achieve potency with the maternal object. At this point, Mr C's initial self-preservative violence is converted to sadomasochistic violence when he makes a conscious and planned decision to kill the man, involving sexual assault on his genitals. This can also be seen as an identifica-tion with the aggressor – the bullied boy becomes the bully, and the murdered man represents a hated image of Mr C as a passive fem-inised figure who must be destroyed.

Dissociation and sexual homicide

For Glasser (1998), as illustrated in this clinical case, sexual homi-cide is a result of the breakdown of sadomasochistic defences to a self-preservative, where the perpetrator becomes threatened by primitive core complex anxieties of engulfment and annihilation and is no longer able to control and torture the object, but instead is driven to eliminate the object altogether in a desperate attempt to preserve their own psychological self. Meloy (2000), however, believes that sexual homicides may be the result of sadomasochistic or predatory violence, where the paraphilic perpetrator's risk of actual violence increases via a fusion of sadistic fantasies with arousal patterns in which the person exhibits "successive approximation" or "behavioural try outs" – engaging in behaviours that bring them progressively closer to the acts they repeatedly fantasise about. By contrast, the psychoanalyst Abby Stein (2004) proposes that crossing the boundary from fantasy into action is not determined by the criminogenic power of the paraphilic fantasy but by the influence of deviant pre-Oedipal object relations and dissociative defences. In her analysis of the confessions of two men who kidnapped, raped, killed, and mutilated a young woman, she explores the role of dissociation and unconscious fantasy in violent and paraphilic sexual offending. Like Glasser, Stein locates the origins of violence in the childhood trauma of perceived psychic obliteration by the maternal object, but she proposes that dissociation, rather than sadomasochistic aggression, is the default defensive position of the sexual offender, whose perverse fantasies and behaviours are defences against the anxiety and ego dissolution of such annihilation. The overtly sexual nature of these fantasies conceals their primary wish for symbiosis and fusion with the object to compensate for the absence of a parental figure who could satisfy the infant's needs in the earliest stages of separation-individuation (Mahler, 1968). The adult perpetrator re-creates this longed for state in his sexual crime by an imagined intimacy with the victim where there are no boundaries between self and other, and active perpetration and active resistance are not differentiated. Dissociative experiences of trauma are reorganised via fantasies of symbiosis and fusion, creating the allusion of sufficiency. Stein proposes that rape fulfils an unconscious fantasy of symbiotic fusion of filling and crawling back inside the womb. However, this closeness triggers the fear of engulfment from which the only escape is murder to reinstate separateness and restore homeostasis.

Treatment considerations

Most available treatments for sex offenders are based on cognitive behavioural principles and are offered in the criminal justice system rather than in health settings, but there is also evidence that multisystemic therapy (MST), an intensive, family-focused, and community-based treatment, as well as therapeutic communities, are effective (Holper et al., 2024).

The treatment of sexual offenders with ASPD present particular difficulties. Compared to sexual offenders without ASPD, they tend to be less internally motivated to engage in treatment or motivated only by external factors such as early release from prison and are more disruptive in group therapy; for example, making inappropriate comments about other group members or undermining the therapists, and they are more likely to minimise or deny their sexual offences (Marshall, 2022). These characteristics create challenges in managing the dynamics in groups with sexual offenders without ASPD. Different problems may be encountered when sexual offenders with ASPD are treated in groups of offenders with ASPD who have violent, but not sexual, offences. In these groups, those patients or offenders whose offending is not sexual may not tolerate those with sexual offences, and these individuals may be scapegoated or excluded from the group. Sexual offending in general is associated with considerable shame, stigma, and alienation from society, but those sexual offenders who have ASPD with significant histories of adverse childhood experiences may be particularly sensitive to these difficulties (Hopton et al., 2021).

Finally, the emotional burden of working with such offenders should not be overestimated. There is some evidence that staff treating this population have higher rates of burnout and even increased mortality (Craissati, 2018), which stresses the importance of clinical supervision and reflective practice in which counter-transference responses and problematic team dynamics may be explored and contained.

Chapter 10

Black lives matter

The criminalisation of blackness

The figures regarding the criminalisation and mass incarceration of black people are stark. Most studies of the demographics of prison populations have been conducted in the United States, but more recent research shows that over-representation of ethnic and racial groups in prisons occurs in all democracies worldwide where such data is collected. This disproportionality occurs not only in countries such as the United States, the United Kingdom, South Africa, Australia, or Brazil, where there are histories of racial oppression, settler colonialism, or significant wealth inequality, but also in countries such as Norway and Germany, where there is fairer wealth distribution and more progressive penal policies. The US and the UK have the highest rates of incarceration of people of African heritage compared to other ethnic groups. In 2024, black or black British individuals made up 12.1% of the prison population, despite constituting only 4.0% of the general population, and more broadly, people from Black, Asian, Minority Ethnic (BAME) backgrounds accounted for 27% of the prison population compared to 13% of the general population.

Individuals with ASPD are also over-represented in offender populations, including prison and probation (Prins, 2014), but exploration of the relationship between ASPD and race has been limited to date (Edwards et al., 2024). A systematic review and meta-analysis of 15 studies examining personality disorders, race, and ethnicity, conducted in a variety of settings in the UK and

DOI: 10.4324/9781003559801-15

US, found that there were no significant differences in the prevalence of personality disorders for Asian or Hispanic groups relative to whites, but black individuals were less likely to have a diagnosis of any personality disorder compared to whites, although studies that looked specifically at ASPD showed no significant difference (McGilloway et al., 2010). A more recent large-scale US population study reported that Native Americans showed a significantly higher lifetime prevalence of ASPD, while Asians/Pacific Islanders and Hispanics showed lower prevalence; and blacks had a similar rate to whites (Goldstein et al., 2017).

Whilst these statistics indicate that black people are no more likely to have ASPD than white people, studies have shown that they are nevertheless treated differently. Compared to their white counterparts, black persons with ASPD are less likely to receive psychiatric care in prison (Coid et al., 2002; Edwards et al., 2024), with one study showing that this is particularly the case for black women (Coid et al., 2002). Black men with symptoms of ASPD and/or psychopathic traits and related characteristics such as anger, aggression, and impulsivity are more likely to be arrested, imprisoned, given harsher sentences, denied bail, and have earlier contact with the criminal justice system than white men showing similar presentations (Brownlow et al., 2024; Edwards et al., 2024; Ehlers et al., 2022; Kovera, 2019; Verona & Fox, 2025). There is also some evidence that in court cases some lawyers deliberately racially misuse antisocial personality disorder and psychopathy labels to prosecute and punish people from black and ethnic minority backgrounds (Argueta-Cevallos, 2021).

Young people are also disproportionally and adversely affected. Racially minoritised, especially black, youths are more often subject to harsh school disciplinary practices that lead to poor educational outcomes and criminal justice involvement than white children (Barnes & Motz, 2018; Marchbanks et al., 2018). In the UK, black individuals are over nine times more likely to be stopped and searched, and BAME people make up half of all prisoners in young offender institutions, despite being a smaller share of the population (Carr, 2017). In a process known as "adultification" black children are more likely to be perceived as older, guilty, and deserving of punishment by white law enforcement agencies compared to white children, depriving them of their innocence (Aiyegbusi, 2023). Black children are also disproportionally subjected to strip searching than their white counterparts (Children's Commissioner, 2023).

Psychoanalysis and racism

Despite the wealth of evidence implicating systemic racism in the criminalisation, incarceration, and homicide of black people, including those with ASPD, meaningful shifts in public attitudes, government policies, or criminal justice system practices to address this remain limited. Compared to other disciplines within the humanities and social sciences, psychoanalysis has arrived late to the table in recognising and exploring issues of race. Its focus on the individual and the internal unconscious world of phantasy has neglected the influence of social, cultural, and political currents in the external world and the legacy of the real historical traumas and their ongoing transgenerational impact.

Freud's universal theory of the human mind divorced from the influence of culture and society, which may have protected him from knowing his own racist experiences as a Jew, stymied psychoanalytic interest in acknowledging and understanding the experiences of the racially oppressed (Stoute, 2021). Those early psychoanalytic writers (e.g. Sterba, 1947) who did consider racism emphasised individual psychopathology in Oedipal conflict and sibling rivalry, where the black man served as displacement object for aggressive and Oedipal conflicts – the cruel powerful father who must be killed (lynched) by the (white) sons (Gordon, 1993).

Frantz Fanon, a black French psychiatrist and political philosopher from the French colony of Martinique, effected a radical shift in psychoanalytic theory on racism by prioritising black subjectivity. Influenced by Sartre and Lacan and exploring his own painful experiences of colonial racism, he demonstrated how the black man's identity is created through the eyes of white people, whose objectification and dehumanisation forges a fundamental split in the psyche, where the black man is alienated from himself and forced to choose between accepting white supremacy or becoming non-existent (Fanon, 1952).

Following Fanon, more recent psychoanalytic explorations of racism have applied Kleinian concepts, identifying pre-Oedipal conflicts and emphasising issues of similarity and difference, anxieties about separation, and the defence mechanisms of splitting, projection, and projective identification (Keval, 2001). The recognition of another person's difference can trigger deep, unconscious anxieties about being separate, which may originate in early infantile experiences of separation from the maternal object, accompanied by anxieties about dependence and the threat of change. The awareness of difference can evoke intense primitive feelings of shame and humiliation, and so to maintain separateness, the person projects unwanted aspects of himself into the other, who becomes the receptacle of his projections. These projections are of infantile or psychotic intensity, and therefore highly resistant to rationality. In racism, visible differences such as skin colour can become a target for attack.

Thus, several authors (Kovel, 1988; Davids, 1992) have suggested that a specific phantasy underlies racist thought: a desire for fusion with the object, where the racist state of mind acts as a hostile strategy to control the object and prevent separation. Keval (2005) characterised the racist state of mind as a pathological defensive organisation of the self or as a form of "psychic retreat" (Steiner, 1993) which functions to shield the individual from overwhelming anxieties linked to experiences of separateness. The historical dynamics of the "master-slave" or "coloniser-colonised" relationship are projected onto the early mother-infant relationship (Keval, 2001). Racism can be seen to exist within a hierarchical or "up-down" framework, where a nurturing, "horizontal" connection to the breast fails and the infant shifts into a "vertical" world defined by power struggles, where experience is polarised into only two possibilities: domination or degradation (Numa, 2023). However, Davids (2006) argues that these conceptualisations rely on the presence of primitive psychic functioning within the racist person associated with individual psychopathology, and do not account for the fact that adults who do not consider themselves racist nevertheless may not intervene when they witness something racist. He suggests that we all contain an internal racist organisation within the mind, – "normal pathological organisation" – which is a normal developmental achievement that becomes available to the individual as a means of managing overwhelming anxiety.

Another crucial question is why racial categories, and specifically gradations of skin colour, should attract these projections. There is now widespread recognition that the concept of race is invalid (Gordon, 1993) – there are no boundaries between human beings based on a biological and genetic basis, and that racism is a social, historical, political, and historical phenomenon. Colourism was the invention of the European colonisers, who established a racial hierarchy and exploited skin colour to rationalise the enslavement and subjugation of Africans and Native Americans. Rustin (1991) has described the category of race as empty and devoid of real meaning and therefore the perfect container for unwanted aspects of the self, expelled via projective identification.

Racism is organised around power and persists to maintain the status quo in systems, organisations, and society. Part of its power is that "whiteness" exists as an organising principle in the unconscious (Dennis, 2020) but is denied and disavowed by liberal white society. However, their unconscious racism is betrayed by their "white fragility" (DiAngelo, 2018), where a minimal racial challenge will trigger anger, shame, guilt, or anxiety, which spurs a retreat into protective insulated spaces and stifles any real efforts to confront the ongoing legacy of colonial supremacy.

The trauma of racism

In his seminal work *Black Skin, White Mask*, Fanon (1952) vividly described the tragic fate of the black man who, through the gaze of the white man and through a process he called "epidermalization", has internalised colonial racist hatred against himself, splitting his mind and imprisoning him in a dismembered and alienated body that disgusts and revolts him. Fanon referred to what he called the "zone of nonbeing", a state of profound alienation, dehumanisation, objectification, and ontological negation – a space outside of humanity as recognised by the white colonial world. The painful paradox of the black person is that his body is hyper-visible to the white gaze, yet his existence is not seen (Nanji-Rowe, 2025).

More recent psychoanalytic writers, particularly in the forensic field, such as Anne Aiyegbusi and Maxine Dennis, have brought to the fore consideration of the trauma of racism in the concept of embodied racism, where racial trauma is biologically encoded in the body. Racial trauma refers to experiences of harm, prejudice, shame, humiliation, and guilt that a person has suffered or witnessed in the form of microaggressions. Interpersonal, institutional, or systemic racism on a constant and cumulative basis has been shown to have significant negative effects on physical health, including diabetes, hypertension, endocrine disorders, and cardiovascular disease, and increases the likelihood of premature death. It is also associated with many mental health disorders including depression, anxiety, post-traumatic stress disorder, substance misuse, and suicidal thoughts and behaviours (Cénat, 2023). Like embodied trauma (Van der Kolk, 2015), racial trauma is stored non-verbally in the body at a primitive sensorimotor level, manifesting in physical sensations, muscle tension, posture, and physiological reactivity, and although it may not be recalled consciously, the body may react to historical trauma as if it is in the present moment, via visceral feelings, dissociation, fight/flight reactions, or chronic pain (Dennis, 2020).

Importantly, like other forms of trauma, racial trauma may also be transmitted intergenerationally – that is, the adverse psychological and physiological effects of racism are passed from one generation to the next via these non-verbal and unconscious processes. The psychoanalyst Vamik Volkan (1988) has written about how groups may be profoundly affected by historical trauma, which influences the development of both individual and group identity to create representations which can be perpetuated from generation to generation in the collective psyche. In this context, social trauma becomes indistinguishable from personal trauma, as individuals unconsciously identify with the suffering of the group.

More recently, drawing on theories of attachment and epigenetics, the psychotherapist Eugene Ellis suggests that fear stemming from the historical legacy of slavery, even when unspoken, is transferred and inherited intergenerationally, priming the black person's autonomic nervous system to be hyperalert and more reactive to threat (Ellis, 2024). This is relevant for individuals with ASPD, who may be already physiologically and emotionally dysregulated due to their individual childhood histories of trauma; for those who are also black and subject to collective historical and current racial traumas, this process may be compounded.

Blackness as badness

It is easy to see how white men's need to split and project aggressive conflicts into the black person is upheld by casting that person as a dangerous criminal, a fantasy of vilification which becomes concretised in their mass incarceration, where prisons become the repositories of unbearable aspects of humanity (Kita, 2019). The punishment of the black person is a displacement for the white person's need to assuage their disavowed guilt.

Fanon gives many examples of the negative stereotypes and fantasies of how the white portray the primitive nature of the black man: he is bad, ignorant, irrational, impulsive, overly emotional, closer to nature, and a beast, which accounts for his sexual voracity and genital potency. Fanon understood the white man's fantasy of the black man's wish to rape the white woman as the splitting and projection of white sexuality. Davids (1996) adds to Fanon's construction by highlighting its inherent violence.

Extrapolating Freud's (1918) theory of the primal scene as the child's perception of parental sexual intercourse as sadomasochistic violence, Aiyegbusi (2023) proposes that the racial archetype "Big, Black and Dangerous" exists as a primal scene of racial trauma involving murderous violence perpetrated to the black body and functions within the black social unconscious as a persistent and pervasive threat. The processes of internalisation of racism and identification with the aggressor may lead the black person to unconsciously identify with the perpetrator role ascribed to them by the white imagination (Dennis, 2020). One way of understanding this is that if a person has been made to believe that their blackness is badness, he or she may feel deserving of punishment, and therefore commit crimes to assuage the guilt of being black – an example of Freud's *Criminals from a Sense of Guilt* (Freud, 1916).

Black rage

The characterisation of black people as hypersexual, over-emotional, criminal, and violent, or the tropes of the "angry black woman" or the black man in need of policing, precludes an understanding of black anger as a natural response to racial trauma inflicted and endured since the time of slavery. The concept of "black rage" was initially conceived by two African American psychiatrists, William Grier and Price Cobbs, in their seminal 1968 book *Black Rage*, written at the time of the assassination of Martin Luther King Junior and the civil rights movement. They sought to apply a psycho-analytic understanding of the desperation, conflicts, and anger of black life at that time. Their construct has been more recently explored within psychoanalysis by writers such as Beverly Stoute and Fembi Nanji-Rowe as a functional response to racial oppression and degradation that is not solely defensively restrictive but can lead to psychic growth.

Stoute (2021) argues for the introduction of the concept of black rage, incorporating a novel application of the conception of moral injury into the lexicon of analytic theory. She notes that the emotional reaction of rage is not conceptualised as an ego defence or adaptational response. She proposes that black rage, as a powerful and essential defensive psychic force, is distinguished from other forms of rage that are solely reactive and dysfunctional, which if suppressed and internalised result in depression, self-destructive behaviour, or suicide, or if directed externally may lead to violence. Black rage, by contrast, is the transformation of reactive rage via the defensive processes of repression and sub-limation into an adaptive mental energy that both protects self-respect and dignity and empowers and liberates the individual towards socially positive outcomes. The emergence of black rage is also governed by a superego which incorporates the collective unconscious accumulation of transgenerational traumas and the knowledge that what is right has been violated. This is experi-enced as a sense of moral injury – that is a trauma resulting from a betrayal of one's moral or ethical code, in this case the violation of the humanity, rights, and protection of the descendants of slaves – which protects the dignity of the racial self.

Influenced by Fanon's zone of nonbeing and applying a Kleinian psychoanalytic framework, Nanji-Rowe (2025) adds to Stoute's conceptualisation of black rage by incorporating the grief and sorrow that she believes are intimately connected to or defended against by black rage. She reframes Klein's depressive position as a psychic process, "perceiving a black part-object to a whole black person" (Nanji-Rowe, 2025, p. 98) and Klein's concept of mourning to think about reparative anti-racist practices. However, unlike the white person whose loss to be mourned is the omnipotence of whiteness, the loss for the black person is of something never experienced – of being or existing – Fanon's zone of nonbeing. The task, therefore, is to be able to live with the loss rather than give it up, as this is not achievable. At the same time, black rage has the capacity to generate self-love as a psychic conversion from a kind of death (nonbeing) to self-awareness, self-worth, and ultimately self-existence. Black rage is therefore life oriented and enhances change and should find a central place within psychoanalysis rather than at its margins.

Clinical considerations

Patients with ASPD who are also black or from other minority ethnic backgrounds may have experienced multiple levels of trauma; like their white counterparts, this will include childhood experiences of abuse or neglect, but in addition they are likely to have been subject to racial trauma at every stage within their developmental trajectory. Because their exposure to racism is ongoing, they may be in a permanent state of hypervigilance and distrust, which will heighten their sensitivity to perceived threats and lower their threshold for reactive or aggressive responses. The difficult task for clinicians or therapists tasked with helping them to reduce violence and other offending behaviours is to recognise and validate their racial experiences but help them distinguish between what is a legitimate affective response from what is destructive to themselves and others – the difference between black rage and more damaging forms of aggression and violence.

The work is further complicated by the inevitable racialisation of the therapeutic relationship. Awareness of one's unconscious racist attitudes – one's internal racism – is hard to achieve. As such beliefs are deemed unacceptable, the mind's censorship may prevent them reaching consciousness, and they may only reveal themselves in bodily or somatic countertransference responses, such as physiological manifestations of anxiety, anger, or disgust. Unconscious racial elements will also form part of the patient's transference to the therapist, which is not solely a projection of the patient's conflicts but also an unconscious response to the internal racism of the therapist. The patient's experience of the therapist dismissing their racial subjectivity may lead to ruptures in treatment, but impasses may also occur when the therapist's internal racism locks into that of the patient's in an unconscious collusion. Exploring this charged area requires, on the part of the therapist, a willingness to admit mistakes and resist retreating into defensive states of white fragility. Further challenges may occur in therapeutic groups and treatments in wider settings, where multiple implicit and explicit racist states of mind interact and impact both patients and staff in manifold respects, as in the following vignette.

> *Dr G, a female forensic psychotherapist, was the therapist for a psychoanalytically- informed treatment group for violent men with a diagnosis of ASPD in a prison wing run on therapeutic community principles. Of eight group members, two were black – Joe, a second-generation Afro-Caribbean man, and Al, who was from Nigeria. The other group members and Dr G were white. Joe was coming to the end of his sentence for assault on his girlfriend and was due to be released into the community in a few weeks' time. By contrast, George, a white man who was serving a long sentence for armed robbery, was not expecting to be considered for release for at least another two years. George had always appeared in awe of Joe and admired him for his sporting achievements prior to being in prison.*
>
> *The group had been discussing the triggers to their violent actions. Joe spoke poignantly of feeling humiliated by his girlfriend's taunts that she did not find him attractive and was reminded of feeling as a child that his mother was perpetually disappointed in him in some way. For the first time, he became tearful in the group. There was a silence, in which Dr G felt*

moved and thought that the other members felt similarly. To her surprise George suddenly accused Joe of faking his tears, that he was trying to disguise the fact that he was a typical black man who excelled at sports but enjoyed beating his wife. Joe became incensed, and turning to Dr G, asked her to intervene and insist that George be asked to leave the group for making racist remarks that were unacceptable as well as illegal. Al, the other black person in the room, tried to mediate by saying that George had recently made other offensive remarks, such as saying to Dr G that he didn't think female therapists were up to working with violent men and accusing another (white) group member of being intellectually arrogant. Al advised Joe not to take George's remarks seriously.

Dr G felt shocked and confused and said that she could not expel someone from the group for an illegal action when everyone in the group was there because they had done illegal things. She said it was important for the group to try to understand why George had felt like attacking Joe and suggested that it was difficult for group members who did not know when they would be released to see others, like Joe, moving on and leaving prison. George nodded to this remark, but Joe remained very angry and said that if George did not leave the group, then he would leave the group, even though his actual release date was a few weeks hence.

Following this session, Dr G reflected on what had happened, and wondered whether, due to her own unconscious racist assumptions, she had minimised the impact of George's racist remark on Joe, by implicitly agreeing with Al that George's insults should not be taken too seriously. Dr G suspected that Al was protecting himself from feeling racially attacked. She also realised that she had instinctively pathologised Joe's aggressive response to George's racist provocations. In the next group meeting, Joe again raised the issue of racism. This time, Dr G more explicitly suggested that George's remarks had been motivated by envy of change as well as not wanting to face the loss of a friend, and that he had chosen his words knowing that they would hurt Joe the most. Dr G went on to say how perhaps Joe, and even Al, felt that others, including herself, could never fully understand what it was like to be so visibly different and therefore open to attack, but perhaps they all could empathise with experiences of feeling different and ostracised, and this seemed to define the mood of the group at the moment, which was threatened by change with one of its members leaving. George then apologised for what he had said to Joe the previous week, and admitted that he was feeling very despondent, ostracised, and alone in prison, having just received a letter from his girlfriend saying she had met someone else.

Therapists' attunement to the subjectivity of antisocial patients with lived experience of suffering racial trauma is critical in facilitating the transformation of harmful aggression and grievance into more healthy expressions of anger without denying the racial wrongs that have been inflicted upon them. This involves a shift from persecutory functioning to one of mourning of loss, but a loss which pays tribute to black rage and the imperative that black lives do matter.

References

Adler, A. (1924). *The practice and theory of individual psychology.* Kegan Paul, Trench, Trubner.

Adshead, G. (2015). Safety in numbers: Therapy-based index offence work in secure psychiatric care. *Psychoanalytic Psychotherapy*, 29(3), 295–310.

Aichhorn, A. (1965 [1925]). *Wayward youth.* Viking Press.

Aiyegbusi, A. (2023). "Big, black, and dangerous": Primal scene of racial trauma? *The International Journal of Forensic Psychotherapy*, 5(1), 1–19.

Alegria, A. A., Blanco, C., Petry, N. M., Skodol, A. E., Liu, S. M., Grant, B., & Hasin, D. (2013). Sex differences in antisocial personality disorder: Results from the National Epidemiological Survey on Alcohol and Related Conditions. *Personality Disorders*, 4(3), 214–222.

Alexander, F. (1930). The neurotic character. *International Journal of Psychoanalysis*, 11, 292–311.

Alexander, F., & Staub, H. (1931). *The criminal, the judge and the public: A psychological analysis.* MacMillan.

APA (American Psychiatric Association). (1952). *Diagnostic and statistical manual of mental disorders* (1st edn.). American Psychiatric Association.

APA (American Psychiatric Association). (1968). *Diagnostic and statistical manual of mental disorders* (2nd edn.). American Psychiatric Association.

APA (American Psychiatric Association). (2013). *Diagnostic and statistical manual of mental disorders* (5th edn.). American Psychiatric Association.

Argueta-Cevallos, G. (2021). A prosecutor with a smoking gun: Examining the weaponization of race, psychopathy, and ASPD labels in capital cases. *Columbia Human Rights Law Review*, 53, 624–662.

Aromäki, A. S., Lindman, R. E., & Eriksson, C. J. (2002). Testosterone, sexuality and antisocial personality in rapists and child molesters: A pilot study. *Psychiatry Research*, 110(3), 239–247.

Barnes, J. C., & Motz, R. T. (2018). Reducing racial inequalities in adulthood arrest by reducing inequalities in school discipline: Evidence from the school-to-prison pipeline. *Developmental Psychology*, 54(12), 2328–2340. doi:10.1037/dev0000613.

Baron-Cohen, S. (1995). *Mindblindness: An essay on autism and theory of mind*. MIT Press.

Bateman, A. W. (2022). Mentalizing and group psychotherapy: A novel treatment for antisocial personality disorder. *American Journal of Psychotherapy*, 75(1), 32–37. doi:10.1176/appi.psychotherapy.20210023.

Bateman, A., Bolton, R., & Fonagy, P. (2013). Antisocial personality disorder: A mentalizing framework. *Focus*, 11(2), 178–186.

Bateman, A., & Fonagy, P. (1999). Effectiveness of partial hospitalization in the treatment of borderline personality disorder: A randomized controlled trial. *The American Journal of Psychiatry*, 156(10), 1563–1569.

Bateman, A., & Fonagy, P. (2001). Treatment of borderline personality disorder with psychoanalytically oriented partial hospitalization: An 18-month follow-up. *The American Journal of Psychiatry*, 158(1), 36–42.

Bateman, A., & Fonagy, P. (2008). Co-morbid antisocial and borderline personality disorders: mentalization-based treatment. *Journal of Clinical Psychology: in session*, 64(2), 181–194.

Bateman, A., & Fonagy, P. (2009). Randomized controlled trial of outpatient mentalization-based treatment versus structured clinical management for borderline personality disorder. *The American Journal of Psychiatry*, 166(12), 1355–1364.

Bateman, A. W., & Fonagy, P. (2012). Mentalization-based treatment of borderline personality disorder. In T. A. Widiger (Ed.), *The Oxford handbook of personality disorders* (pp. 767–784). Oxford University Press.

Bateman, A., & Fonagy, P. (2016). *Mentalization-based treatment for personality disorders: A practical guide*. Oxford University Press.

Bateman, A., & Fonagy, P. (2019). *Handbook of mentalizing in mental health practice*. American Psychiatric Association Publishing.

Bateman, A., Yakeley, J., & Motz, A. (2019). Mentalizing and antisocial personality disorder. In A. Bateman & P. Fonagy (Eds.), *Handbook of mentalizing in mental health practice* (2nd edn., pp. 335–350). American Psychiatric Association Publishing.

Beech, A. R., & Ward, T. (2004). The integration of etiology and risk in sexual offenders: A theoretical framework. *Aggression and Violent Behavior*, 10(1), 31–63.

Bender, L. (1947). Psychopathic behavior disorders in children. In M. Lindner & R. V. Selinger (Eds.), *Handbook of correctional psychology*. Philosophical Library.

Bion, W. R. (1962). *Learning from experience*. Karnac Books.

Blackburn, B. (1998). Psychopathy and personality disorder: Implications of interpersonal theory. In D. Cooke, A. Forth & R. Hare (Eds.), *Psychopathy: Theory, research and implications for society* (pp. 269–302). Kluwer.

Blair, R. J. R. (1999). Responsiveness to distress cues in the child with psychopathic tendencies. *Personality and Individual Differences*, 27(1), 135–145.

Bloom, B. E., Owen, B., & Covington, S. S. (2005). *Gender-responsive strategies: Research, practice, and guiding principles for women offenders*. National Institute of Corrections. https://nicic.gov/gender-responsive-strategies-research-practice-and-guiding-principles-women-offenders.

Blumenthal, S., Huckle, C., Czornyj, R., Craissati, J., & Richardson, P. (2010). The role of affect in the estimation of risk. *Journal of Mental Health*, 19(5), 444–451.

Bowlby, J. (1944). Forty-four juvenile thieves: Their characters and home-life (II). *International Journal of Psycho-Analysis*, 25, 107–128.

Bowlby, J. (1969). *Attachment and loss: Vol. 1. Attachment* (2nd edn.). Basic Books.

Bowlby, J. (1973). *Attachment and loss: Vol. 2. Separation: Anxiety and anger*. Basic Books.

Brownlow, B. N., Harmon, K. S., Pek, J., Cheavens, J. S., Moore, J. L., III, & Coccaro, E. F. (2024). Criminalizing psychopathology in Black Americans: Racial and gender differences in the relationship between psychopathology and arrests. *Clinical Psychological Science*, 12(6), 1075–1093.

Cannon, C., Hamel, J., Buttell, F. P., & Ferreira, R. (2016). A survey of domestic violence perpetrator programs in the United States and Canada: Findings and implications for policy and intervention. *Partner Abuse*, 7(3), 226–276.

Carr, N. (2017). The Lammy Review and race and bias in the criminal justice system. *Probation Journal*, 64(4), 333–336.

Cartwright, D. (2002). *Psychoanalysis, violence and rage-type murder*. Brunner-Routledge.

Cénat J. M. (2023). Complex racial trauma: Evidence, theory, assessment, and treatment. *Perspectives on Psychological Science: A Journal of the Association for Psychological Science*, 18(3), 675–687.

Chasseguet-Smirgel, J. (1984). *Creativity and perversion*. W. W. Norton.

Children's Commissioner. (2023). *Strip-searching of children in England and Wales – Analysis by the Children's Commissioner for England*. https://assets.childrenscommissioner.gov.uk/wpuploads/2023/03/cc-strip-search-of-children-in-england-and-wales.pdf.

Choy, O., & Raine, A. (2024). The neurobiology of antisocial personality disorder. *Neuropharmacology*, 261, 110150.

Cleckley, H. (1941). *The mask of sanity.* C. V. Mosby.

Coid, J., Petruckevitch, A., Bebbington, P., Brugha, T., Bhugra, D., Jenkins, R., Farrell, M., Lewis, G., & Singleton, N. (2002). Ethnic differences in prisoners. 1: Criminality and psychiatric morbidity. *The British Journal of Psychiatry,* 181, 473–480.

Coid, J., Yang, M., Ullrich, S., Roberts, A., Moran, P., Bebbington, P., Brugha, T., Jenkins, R., Farrell, M., Lewis, G., Singleton, N., & Hare, R. (2009). Psychopathy among prisoners in England and Wales. *International Journal of Law and Psychiatry,* 32(3), 134–141.

Compton, W. M., Conway, K. P., Stinson, F. S., Colliver, J. D., & Grant, B. F. (2005). Prevalence, correlates, and comorbidity of DSM-IV antisocial personality syndromes and alcohol and specific drug use disorders in the United States: Results from the National Epidemiologic Survey on Alcohol and Related Conditions. *The Journal of Clinical Psychiatry,* 66(6), 677–685.

Cornell, D., Warren, J., Hawk, G., Stafford, E., Oram, G., & Pine, D. (1996). Psychopathy in instrumental and reactive violent offenders. *Journal of Consulting and Clinical Psychology,* 64, 783–790.

Craissati, J. (2018). *The rehabilitation of sexual offenders: Complexity, risk and desistance.* Routledge.

Cunliffe, T. B., Gacono, C. B., Meloy, J. R., & Taylor, E. E. (2013). Are male and female psychopaths equivalent? A Rorschach study. In J. Helfgott (Ed.), *Criminal psychology* (Vol. 2, pp. 423–460). Praeger Publishers.

Dargis, M., Newman, J., & Koenigs, M. (2016). Clarifying the link between childhood abuse history and psychopathic traits in adult criminal offenders. *Personality disorders,* 7(3), 221–228.

Davids, M. F. (1992). The cutting edge of racism: An object relations view. *Bulletin of the British Psycho-Analytical Society,* 28(11), 1–13.

Davids, M. F. (1996). Frantz Fanon: The struggle for inner freedom. *Free Associations,* 6, 205–234.

Davids, M. F. (2006). Internal racism, anxiety and the world outside: Islamophobia post-9/111. *Organizational and Social Dynamics,* 6, 63–85.

De Brito, S. A., & Hodgins, S. (2009). Antisocial personality disorder. In M. McMurran & R. Howard (Eds.), *Personality, personality disorder and violence* (pp. 133–153). Wiley.

DeMause, L. (1990). The history of child assault. *Journal of Psychohistory,* 18(1), 1–29.

Dennis, M. (2020). The criminalisation of blackness. In A. Motz, A. Aiyegbusi, & M. Dennis *Invisible trauma: Women, difference and the criminal justice system* (pp. 33–53). Routledge.

Department of Health & Home Office. (1999). *Managing dangerous people with severe personality disorder: Proposals for policy development*. Home Office and Department of Health.

Deutsch, H. (1934). Über einen Typus der Pseudoaffektivität ⊠„Als ob"⊠. *Internationale Zeitschrift für Psychoanalyse*, 20: 323–335.

Deutsch, H. (1955). The imposter: Contribution to the ego psychology of a type of psychopath. *Psychoanalytic Quarterly*, 24(3), 301–321.

DiAngelo, R. (2018). *White fragility: Why it's so hard for white people to talk about racism*. Beacon Press.

Douglas, K. S., Hart, S. D., Webster, C. D., & Belfrage, H. (2013). *HCR-20V3: Assessing risk for violence – User guide*. Mental Health, Law, and Policy Institute, Simon Fraser University.

Edwards, E. R., Epshteyn, G., Diehl, C. K., Ruiz, D., Coolidge, B., Weiss, N. H., & Stein, L. (2024). Prison or treatment? Gender, racial, and ethnic inequities in mental health care utilization and criminal justice history among incarcerated persons with borderline and antisocial personality disorders. *Law and Human Behavior*, 48(2), 104–116.

Ehlers, C. L., Schuckit, M. A., Hesselbrock, V., Gilder, D. A., Wills, D., & Bucholz, K. (2022). The clinical course of antisocial behaviors in men and women of three racial groups. *Journal of Psychiatric Research*, 151, 319–327.

Eichelman, B. (1988). Toward a rational pharmacotherapy for aggressive and violent behavior. *Hospital and Community Psychiatry*, 1, 31–39.

Ellis, E. (2024). *Transforming race conversations: A healing guide for us all*. W. W. Norton & Co.

Fanon, F. (1952). *Black skin, white masks*. Penguin Random House.

Farrington, D. P., Coid, J. W., Harnett, L., Jolliffe, D., Soteriou, N., Turner, R., & West, D. J. (2006). *Criminal careers up to age 50 and life success up to age 48: New findings from the Cambridge Study in Delinquent Development* (Home Office Research Study No. 299). Home Office.

Fazel, S., & Danesh, J. (2002). Serious mental disorder in 23,000 prisoners: A systematic review of 62 surveys. *The Lancet*, 359(9306), 545–550.

Federn, P. (1913). Beiträge zur Analyse des Sadismus und Masochismus: I. Die Quellen des männlichen Sadismus. *Internationale Zeitschrift für Ärztliche Psychoanalyse*, 1, 29–49.

Federn, P. (1919). *Zur Psychologie der Revolution: Die Vaterlose Gesellschaft. Nach Vorträgen in der Wiener Psychoanalytischen Vereinigung und im Monistenbund*. Anzengruber-Verlag Brüder Suschitzky.

Fenichel, O. (1931). The pre-genital antecedents of the Oedipus complex. *International Journal of Psycho-Analysis*, 12, 412–430.

Fenichel, O. (1945). *The psychoanalytic theory of neurosis*. W. W. Norton.

Ferenczi, S. (1919). Pszichoanalízis és kriminológia. In *A pszichoanalízis haladása: Értekezések* (pp. 126–128). Dick Manó Kiadása.

Ferenczi, S. (1994 [1933]). Confusion of tongues between adults and the child—The language of tenderness and of passion. In *Final contributions to the problems and methods of psychoanalysis* (pp. 156–167). Karnac.

Fonagy, P., & Bateman, A. W. (2006). Mechanisms of change in mentalization-based treatment of BPD. Journal of Clinical Psychology, 62(4), 411–430.

Fonagy, P., Luyten, P., & Allison, E. (2015). Epistemic petrification and the restoration of epistemic trust: A new conceptualization of borderline personality disorder and its psychosocial treatment. *Journal of Personality Disorders*, 29(5), 575–609.

Fonagy, P., Simes, E., Yirmiya, K., Wason, J., Barrett, B., Frater, A., Cameron, A., Butler, S., Hoare, Z., McMurran, M., Moran, P., Crawford, M., Pilling, S., Allison, E., Yakeley, J., & Bateman, A. (2025). Mentalisation-based treatment for antisocial personality disorder in males convicted of an offence on community probation in England and Wales (Mentalization for Offending Adult Males, MOAM): a multicentre, assessor blinded, randomised controlled trial. *The Lancet Psychiatry*, 12 (3), 208–219.

Fontao, M. I., Pfäfflin, F., & Lamott, F. (2006). Application of transference focused psychotherapy (TFP) in forensic-psychiatric inpatients: A pilot study. *Recht und Psychiatrie*, 24(4), 193–200.

Forouzan, E., & Cooke, D. J. (2005). Figuring out la femme fatale: Conceptual and assessment issues concerning psychopathy in females. *Behavioral Sciences & the Law*, 23(6), 765–778.

Foulkes, S. H. (1983 [1948]). *Introduction to group-analytic psychotherapy.* Karnac Books.

Francia, C., Coolidge, F., White, L., Segal, D., Cahill, B., & Estey, A. (2010). Personality disorder profiles in incarcerated male rapists and child molesters. *American Journal of Forensic Psychology*, 28, 1–14.

Freud, A. (1966 [1936]). *The ego and the mechanisms of defense.* International Universities Press.

Freud, A. (1947). Certain types and stages of social maladjustment. In *The writings of Anna Freud: Indications for child analysis and other papers, 1945–1956* (Vol. 3, pp. 75–94), International Universities Press.

Freud, S. (1905). *Three essays on the theory of sexuality.* In J. Strachey (Ed. & Trans.), The standard edition of the complete psychological works of Sigmund Freud (Vol. 7, pp. 123–245). Hogarth Press and the Institute of Psychoanalysis.

Freud, S. (1906). *Psycho-analysis and the establishment of the facts in legal proceedings.* In J. Strachey (Ed. & Trans.), The standard edition of the complete psychological works of Sigmund Freud (Vol. 9, pp. 97–114). Hogarth Press.

Freud, S. (1913). *Totem and taboo: Some points of agreement between the mental lives of savages and neurotics* (J. Strachey, Trans.). In J. Strachey (Ed. & Trans.), The standard edition of the complete psychological works of Sigmund Freud (Vol. 13, pp. 1–161). Hogarth Press.

Freud, S. (1914). *Remembering, repeating and working-through (Further recommendations on the technique of psycho-analysis II).* In J. Strachey (Ed. & Trans.), The standard edition of the complete psychological works of Sigmund Freud (Vol. 12, pp. 145–156). Hogarth Press.

Freud, S. (1916). *Some character-types met with in psycho-analytic work: III. Criminals from a sense of guilt.* In J. Strachey (Ed. & Trans.), The standard edition of the complete psychological works of Sigmund Freud (Vol. 14, pp. 309–333). Hogarth Press.

Freud, S. (1918). *From the history of an infantile neurosis.* In J. Strachey (Ed. & Trans.), The standard edition of the complete psychological works of Sigmund Freud (Vol. 17, pp. 1–124). Hogarth Press.

Freud, S. (1920). *Beyond the pleasure principle.* In J. Strachey (Ed. & Trans.), The standard edition of the complete psychological works of Sigmund Freud (Vol. 18, pp. 1–64). Hogarth Press.

Freud, S. (1923). *The ego and the id.* In J. Strachey (Ed. & Trans.), The standard edition of the complete psychological works of Sigmund Freud (Vol. 19, pp. 12–66). Hogarth Press.

Freud, S. (1924). *The economic problem of masochism.* In J. Strachey (Ed. & Trans.), The standard edition of the complete psychological works of Sigmund Freud (Vol. 19, pp. 155–170). Hogarth Press.

Freud, S. (1927). *Fetishism.* In J. Strachey (Ed. & Trans.), The standard edition of the complete psychological works of Sigmund Freud (Vol. 21, pp. 149–157). Hogarth Press.

Freud, S. (1928). *Dostoevsky and parricide.* In J. Strachey (Ed. & Trans.), The standard edition of the complete psychological works of Sigmund Freud (Vol. 21, pp. 173–194). Hogarth Press.

Freud, S. (1930). *Civilisation and its discontents.* In J. Strachey (Ed. & Trans.), The standard edition of the complete psychological works of Sigmund Freud (Vol. 21, pp. 57–146). Hogarth Press.

Freud, S. (1938). *Splitting of the ego in the process of defence.* In J. Strachey (Ed. & Trans.), The standard edition of the complete psychological works of Sigmund Freud (Vol. 23, pp. 271–278). Hogarth Press.

Frick, P. J., Cornell, A. H., Bodin, S. D., Dane, H. E., Barry, C. T., & Loney, B. R. (2003). Callous-unemotional traits and developmental pathways to severe conduct problems. *Developmental Psychology*, 39(2), 246–260.

Friedlander, K. (1947). *The psychoanalytic approach to juvenile delinquency.* Routledge.

Frodi, A., Dernevik, M., Sepa, A., Philipson, J., & Bragesjö, M. (2001). Current attachment representations of incarcerated offenders varying in degree of psychopathy. *Attachment & Human Development*, 3(3), 269–283.

Fromm, E. (1964). *The heart of man: Its genius for good and evil.* Lantern Books.

Gabbard, G. O. (2005). *Psychodynamic psychiatry in clinical practice: The DSM-IV edition.* American Psychiatric Press.

Gabbard, G. O., & Coyne, L. (1987). Predictors of response of antisocial patients to hospital treatment. *Hospital and Community Psychiatry*, 38(11), 1181–1185.

Gacono, C. B., & Meloy, J. R. (1991). A Rorschach investigation of attachment and anxiety in antisocial personality disorder. *Journal of Nervous and Mental Disease*, 179(9), 546 552.

Gacono, C. B., & Meloy, J. R. (1994). *The Rorschach assessment of aggressive and psychopathic personalities.* Erlbaum.

Gacono, C. B., & Smith, J. M. (2021). Understanding the psychopath from a psychodynamic perspective: A Rorschach study. *Archives of Assessment Psychology*, 11, Article 7.

George, C., Kaplan, N., & Main, M. (1996). Adult attachment interview. Unpublished manuscript, University of California, Berkeley.

Gibbon, S., Duggan, C., Stoffers, J., Huband, N., Völlm, B. A., Ferriter, M., & Lieb, K. (2010). Psychological interventions for antisocial personality disorder. *Cochrane Database of Systematic Reviews*, 6, Article CD007668.

Gibbon, S., Khalifa, N. R., Cheung, N. H. Y., Völlm, B. A., & McCarthy, L. (2020). Psychological interventions for antisocial personality disorder. *Cochrane Database of Systematic Reviews*, 9, Article CD007668.

Gilligan, J. (1996). *Violence: Our deadliest epidemic and its causes.* Grosset/Putnam.

Glasser, M. (1986). Identification and its vicissitudes as observed in the perversions. *International Journal of Psycho-Analysis*, 67, 9–17.

Glasser, M. (1996). Aggression and sadism in the perversions. In I. Rosen (Ed.), *Sexual deviation* (3rd edn.). Oxford University Press.

Glasser, M. (1998). On violence: A preliminary communication. *International Journal of Psycho-Analysis*, 79, 887–902.

Goldstein, R. B., Chou, S. P., Saha, T. D., Smith, S. M., Jung, J., Zhang, H., Pickering, R. P., Ruan, W. J., Huang, B., & Grant, B. F. (2017). The epidemiology of antisocial behavioral syndromes in adulthood: Results from the National Epidemiologic Survey on Alcohol and Related Conditions-III. *The Journal of Clinical Psychiatry*, 78(1), 90–98.

Goodwin, R. D., & Hamilton, S. P. (2003). Lifetime comorbidity of antisocial personality disorder and anxiety disorders among adults in the community. *Psychiatry Research*, 117(2), 159–166.

Gordon, P. (1993). Souls in armour: Thoughts on psychoanalysis and racism. *British Journal of Psychotherapy*, 10(1), 62–76.

Greenacre, P. (1945). Conscience in the psychopath. *American Journal of Orthopsychiatry*, 15(3), 495–509.

Greenacre, P. (1958). The imposter. *Psychoanalytic Quarterly*, 27, 359–383.

Greenfeld, L. A., & Snell, T. L. (1999). *Women offenders* (Bureau of Justice Statistics Bulletin). U.S. Department of Justice.

Grier, W. H., & Cobbs, P. M. (1968). *Black rage.* Basic Books.

Hanson, R. K., & Morton-Bourgon, K. E. (2005). The characteristics of persistent sexual offenders: A meta-analysis of recidivism studies. *Journal of Consulting and Clinical Psychology*, 73(6), 1154–1163.

Hare, R. (1991). *Manual of the revised psychopathy checklist.* Multi Health Systems.

Hare, R. (2003). *Hare psychopathy checklist—Revised (PCL-R): 2nd edition technical manual.* Multi-Health Systems.

Hare, R. D., & Thorvaldson, S. A. (1970). Psychopathy and response to electrical stimulation. *Journal of Abnormal Psychology*, 76(3, Pt.1), 370–374.

Harlow, H. F., Dodsworth, R. O., & Harlow, M. K. (1965). Total social isolation in monkeys. *Proceedings of the National Academy of Sciences of the United States of America*, 54(1), 90–97.

Harris, G. T., Rice, M. E., & Cormier, C. A. (1994). Psychopaths: Is a therapeutic community therapeutic? *Therapeutic Communities*, 15, 283–299.

Healy, W. (1915). *The individual delinquent: A text-book of diagnosis and prognosis for all concerned in understanding offenders.* Little, Brown, and Company.

Holper, L., Mokros, A., & Habermeyer, E. (2024). Moderators of sexual recidivism as indicators of treatment effectiveness in persons with sexual offence histories: An updated meta-analysis. *Sexual Abuse*, 26(3), 255–291.

Hopton, J., Van Gerko, K., Ashworth, J., & Craissati, J. (2021). Exploring preliminary outcomes of a community treatment programme for men with sexual convictions screened into the offender personality disorder pathway. *The Journal of Forensic Psychiatry & Psychology*, 32(2), 226–241.

Horney, K. (1945). *Our inner conflicts: A constructive theory of neurosis.* W. W. Norton.

Houser, M. C. (2015). A history of antisocial personality disorder in the diagnostic and statistical manual of mental illness and treatment from a rehabilitation perspective. Dissertation.

Howell, E. F. (2014). Ferenczi's concept of identification with the aggressor: Understanding dissociative structure with interacting victim and abuser self-states. *American Journal of Psychoanalysis,* 74(1), 48–59.

Howell, E. F. (2018). Outsiders to love: The psychopathic character and dilemma. *Contemporary Psychoanalysis,* 54(1), 17–39.

Hyde, L. W., Waller, R., Trentacosta, C. J., Shaw, D. S., Neiderhiser, J. M., Ganiban, J. M., Reiss, D., & Leve, L. D. (2016). Heritable and nonheritable pathways to early callous-unemotional behaviors. *The American Journal of Psychiatry,* 173(9), 903–910.

Jacobson, E. (1964). *The self and the object world.* International University Press.

Jacobson, E. (1971). *Depression.* International University Press.

Jones, M. (1952). *A study of therapeutic communities.* Tavistock.

Joseph, N., & Benefield, N. (2012). A joint offender personality disorder pathway strategy: an outline summary. *Criminal Behaviour and Mental Health,* 22(3), 210–217.

Karpman, B. (1946). Psychopathy in the scheme of human typology. *Journal of Nervous and Mental Disease,* 103(3), 276–288.

Kernberg, O. F. (1976). *Object relations theory and clinical psychoanalysis.* Jason Aronson.

Kernberg, O. F. (1984). *Severe personality disorders.* Yale University Press.

Keval, N. (2001). Understanding the trauma of racial violence in a black patient. *British Journal of Psychotherapy,* 18, 34–51.

Keval, N. (2005). Racist states of mind: An attack on thinking and curiosity. In M. Bower (Ed.), *Psychoanalytic ideas for social work practice: Thinking under fire* (pp. 31–43). Routledge.

Kimonis, E. R., Frick, P. J., Fazekas, H., & Loney, B. R. (2006). Psychopathy, aggression, and the processing of emotional stimuli in non-referred girls and boys. *Behavioral Sciences & the Law,* 24(1), 21–37.

Kita, E. (2019). "They hate me now but where was everyone when I needed them?": Mass incarceration, projective identification, and social work praxis. *Psychoanalytic Social Work,* 26(1), 25–49.

Klein, M. (1927). Criminal tendencies in normal children. *British Journal of Medical Psychology,* 7(2), 177–192.

Klein, M. (1934). On criminality. *The International Journal of Psychoanalysis,* 15, 125–131.

Klein, M. (1964). *Contributions to psychoanalysis: 1920–1945*. McGraw Hill.

Klein, M. (1975 [1946]). Notes on some schizoid mechanisms. In *Envy and gratitude and other works*. Hogarth.

Klein, M. (1975 [1957]). Envy and gratitude. In *Envy and gratitude and other works*. Hogarth.

Kohut, H. (1971). *The analysis of the self: A systematic approach to the psychoanalytic treatment of narcissistic personality disorders*. The University of Chicago Press.

Kolla, N. J., Malcolm, C., Attard, S., Arenovich, T., Blackwood, N., & Hodgins, S. (2013). Childhood maltreatment and aggressive behaviour in violent offenders with psychopathy. *Canadian Journal of Psychiatry/ Revue canadienne de psychiatrie*, 58(8), 487–494.

Kovel, J. (1988). *White racism: A psychohistory*. Free Association Books.

Kovera, M. B. (2019). Racial disparities in the criminal justice system: Prevalence, causes, and a search for solutions. *Journal of Social Issues*, 75(4), 1139–1164.

Lenzenweger, M. F., Lane, M. C., Loranger, A. W., & Kessler, R. C. (2007). DSM-IV personality disorders in the National Comorbidity Survey Replication. *Biological Psychiatry*, 62(5), 553–564.

Levinson, A., & Fonagy, P. (2004). Offending and attachment: The relationship between interpersonal awareness and offending in a prison population with psychiatric disorder. *Canadian Journal of Psychoanalysis*, 12, 225–251.

Levy, D. M. (1937). Primary affect hunger. *The American Journal of Psychiatry*, 94, 643–652.

Linehan, M. M. (1993). *Cognitive-behavioural treatment of borderline personality disorder*. Guilford Press.

Lombroso, C. (1911 [1876]). *Criminal man: According to the classification of Cesare Lombroso*. The Knickerbocker Press.

Loucks, A. (1995). Criminal behavior, violent behavior, and prison maladjustment in federal female offenders. Unpublished doctoral dissertation, Queen's University, Kingston, Canada.

Lykken, D. T. (1957). A study of anxiety in the sociopathic personality. *Journal of Abnormal and Social Psychology*, 55(1), 6–10.

Mahler, M. S. (1968). *On human symbiosis and the vicissitudes of individuation. Vol. I. Infantile psychosis*. International Universities Press.

Mahler, M. S. (1979). *Selected papers of Margaret S. Mahler*. Jason Aronson.

Marchbanks, M. P., III, Peguero, A. A., Varela, K. S., Blake, J. J., & Eason, J. M. (2018). School strictness and disproportionate minority contact: Investigating racial and ethnic disparities with the "school-to-prison pipeline". *Youth Violence and Juvenile Justice*, 16(2), 241–259.

Marshall, L. E. (2022). The antisocial sex offender. In D. W. Black & N. J. Kolla (Eds.), *Textbook of antisocial personality disorder* (pp. 461–476). American Psychiatric Association Publishing.

Marshall, L., & Cooke, D. (1999). The childhood experiences of psychopaths: A retrospective study of familial and societal factors. *Journal of Personality Disorders*, 13, 211–225.

Marshall, W. L., & Marshall, L. E. (2000). The origins of sexual offending. *Trauma, Violence, & Abuse*, 1(3), 250–263.

Maxwell-Scott, G. (2021). A banging door, a gâteau and a knife: Antisocial to prosocial constellations in a forensic group for men. *British Journal of Psychotherapy*, 37(4), 579–593.

McEllistrem, J. (2004). Affective and predatory violence: A bimodal classification system of human aggression and violence. *Aggression and Violent Behavior*, 10, 1–30.

McGauley, G., Adshead, G., & Sarkar, S. (2007). Psychotherapy of psychopathic disorders. In A. Felthouse & H. Sass (Eds.), *The international handbook of psychopathic disorders and the law: Diagnosis and treatment* (Vol. 1, pp. 449–466). John Wiley & Sons.

McGilloway, A., Hall, R. E., Lee, T., & Bhui, K. S. (2010). A systematic review of personality disorder, race and ethnicity: Prevalence, aetiology and treatment. *BMC Psychiatry*, 10(1), Article 33.

McGuire, J. (2022). Psychosocial treatment of antisocial personality disorder. In D. W. Black & N. J. Kolla (Eds.), *Textbook of antisocial personality disorder* (pp. 349–373). American Psychiatric Association Publishing.

Meloy, J. R. (1988). *The psychopathic mind: Origins, dynamics and treatment*. Jason Aronson.

Meloy, J. R. (1992). *Violent attachments*. Jason Aronson.

Meloy, J. R. (2000). The nature and dynamics of sexual homicide: An integrative review. *Aggression and Violent Behavior*, 5(1), 1–22.

Meloy, J. R. (2006). The empirical basis and forensic application of affective and predatory violence. *Australian & New Zealand Journal of Psychiatry*, 40(6–7), 539–547.

Meloy, J. R., & Meloy, M. J. (2003). Autonomic arousal in the presence of psychopathy: A survey of mental health and criminal justice professionals. *Journal of Threat Assessment*, 2(2), 21–33.

Meloy, J. R., & Yakeley, J. (2010). Treatment of cluster B disorders: Antisocial personality disorder. In J. Clarkin, P. Fonagy, & G. Gabbard (Eds.), *Psychodynamic psychotherapy for personality disorders: A clinical handbook* (pp. 349–378). American Psychiatric Publishing.

Meloy, J. R., & Yakeley, J. (2013). Antisocial personality disorder. In G. O. Gabbard & J. Gunderson (Eds.), *Gabbard's treatments of psychiatric disorders* (5th edn.). American Psychiatric Publishing.

Money-Kyrle, R. (1971). The aim of psychoanalysis. *The International Journal of Psycho-Analysis*, 52(1), 103–106.

Morel, B. A. (1857). *Traité des dégénérescences physiques, intellectuelles et morales de l'espèce humaine et des causes qui produisent ces variétés maladives.* J.-B. Baillière.

Motz, A. (2008). *The psychology of female violence: Crimes against the body* (2nd edn.). Routledge.

Nanji-Rowe, F. (2025). Black rage, white gaze: How can black lives, historically reified, have 'room to breathe' in contemporary psychoanalysis? *British Journal of Psychotherapy*, 41(1), 88–105.

Numa, S. (2023). How psychoanalysis can contribute to understanding racism. *The International Journal of Psycho-Analysis*, 104(5), 860–868.

Ogloff, J. R. P., Wong, S., & Greenwood, A. (1990). Treating criminal psychopaths in a therapeutic community program. *Behavioural Sciences and the Law*, 8(2), 181–190.

Oronowicz-Jaśkowiak, W., Lew-Starowicz, M., & Markuszewski, L. (2024). Comparison of risk of recidivism among sexual offenders with and without sexual preference disorders using the STATIC-99R instrument. *Postępy Psychiatrii i Neurologii*, 33(1), 9–17.

Özel, B., Karakaya, E., Köksal, F., Altinoz, A. E., & Yilmaz-Karaman, I. G. (2025). Gender bias of antisocial and borderline personality disorders among psychiatrists. *Archives of Women's Mental Health*, 28, 563–571.

Papagathonikou, T., & Marono, A. (2025). The relationship between psychopathy and sexual sadism: A mixed-methods study. *Journal of Forensic Psychiatry & Psychology*, 36(3), 407–429.

Patrick, C. J. (2018). Cognitive and emotional processing in psychopathy. In C. J. Patrick (Ed.), *Handbook of psychopathy* (pp. 422–455). The Guilford Press.

Pinel, P. (1806). *A treatise on insanity.* Messers Cadell & Davies.

Prichard, J.C. (1835). *A treatise on insanity and other disorders affecting the mind.* Sherwood, Gilbert and Piper.

Prins, S. J. (2014). Prevalence of mental illnesses in U.S. state prisons: A systematic review. *Psychiatric Services*, 65(7), 862–872. doi:10.1176/appi.ps.201300166.

Reich, W. (1945). *Character analysis* (2nd edn.). Farrar, Strauss and Giroux.

Reik, T. (1925). *Geständniszwang und Strafbedürfnis: Probleme der Psychoanalyse und der Kriminologie.* Internationaler Psychoanalytischer Verlag.

Reik, T. (1932). *Der unbekannte Mörder: Von der Tat zum Täter*. Internationaler Psychoanalytischer Verlag.

Rice, M. E., Harris, G. T., & Lang, C. (2013). Validation of and revision to the VRAG and SORAG: The Violence Risk Appraisal Guide—Revised (VRAG-R). *Psychological Assessment, 25*(3), 951–965.

Richards, H. (1998). Evil intent: Violence and disorders of the will. In T. Millon, E. Simonson, M. Birket-Smith, & R. D. Davis (Eds.), *Psychopathy: Antisocial, criminal and violent behavior* (pp. 69–94). The Guilford Press.

Rogstad, J. E., & Rogers, R. (2008). Gender differences in contributions of emotion to psychopathy and antisocial personality disorder. *Clinical Psychology Review, 28*(8), 1472–1484.

Rush, B. (1812). *Medical inquiries and observations upon the diseases of the mind*. Kimber & Richardson.

Rustin, M. (1991). Psychoanalysis, racism and anti-racism. In *The good society and the inner world: Psychoanalysis, politics and culture*. Verso.

Saville, E., & Rumney, D. (1992). *"Let justice be done!": A history of the ISTD*. Institute for the Study and Treatment of Delinquency.

Schlapobersky, J. (1996). A group-analytic perspective: From the speech of hands to the language of words. In C. Cordess & M. Cox (Eds.), *Forensic psychotherapy: Crime, psychodynamics and the offender patient* (pp. 227–243). Jessica Kingsley.

Schmideberg, M. (1935). The psycho-analysis of asocial children and adolescents. *International Journal of Psycho-Analysis, 16*(6), 22–48.

Sevecke, K., Franke, S., Kosson, D., & Krischer, M. (2016). Emotional dysregulation and trauma predicting psychopathy dimensions in female and male juvenile offenders. *Child and Adolescent Psychiatry and Mental Health, 10*, 43.

Siegel, A., & Victoroff, J. (2009). Understanding human aggression: New insights from neuroscience. *International Journal of Law and Psychiatry, 32*, 209–215.

Simonsen, E. (2022). Antisocial personality disorder throughout time: Evolution of the disorder. In D. W. Black & N. J. Kolla (Eds.), *Textbook of antisocial personality disorder* (pp. 15–25). American Psychiatric Association Publishing.

Smith, J. M., Gacono, C. B., Cunliffe, T. B., Kivisto, A. J., & Taylor, E. E. (2014). Psychodynamics in the female psychopath: A PCL-R/Rorschach investigation. *Violence and Gender, 1*(4), 176–187.

Stein, A. (2004). Fantasy, fusion, and sexual homicide. *Contemporary Psychoanalysis, 40*(4), 495–517.

Steiner, J. (1993). *Psychic retreats: Pathological organizations in neurotic, psychotic and borderline patients*. New Library of Psychoanalysis.

Sterba, R. (1947). Some psychological factors in Negro race hatred and in anti-Negro riots. In G. Róheim (Ed.), *Psychoanalysis and the social sciences* (pp. 411–427). International Universities Press.

Stoller, R. J. (1974). Hostility and mystery in perversion. *International Journal of Psycho-Analysis*, 55, 425–434.

Stoller, R. J. (1975). *Perversion*. Pantheon.

Stoute, B. J. (2021). Black rage: The psychic adaptation to the trauma of oppression. *Journal of the American Psychoanalytic Association*, 69(2), 259–290.

Svrakic, D., McCallum, K., & Milan, P. (1991). Developmental, structural and clinical approach to narcissistic and antisocial personalities. *American Journal of Psychoanalysis*, 51, 413–432.

Symington, N. (1980). The response aroused by the psychopath. *International Review of Psychoanalysis*, 7(3), 291–298.

Taubner, S., White, L. O., Zimmermann, J., Fonagy, P., & Nolte, T. (2012). Mentalization moderates and mediates the link between psychopathy and aggressive behavior in male adolescents. *Journal of the American Psychoanalytic Association*, 60, 605–612.

Van der Kolk, B. (2015). *The body keeps the score: Brain, mind, and body in the healing of trauma*. Penguin.

van der Zouwen, M., Hoeve, M., Hendriks, A. M., Asscher, J. J., & Stams, G. J. J. M. (2018). The association between attachment and psychopathic traits. *Aggression and Violent Behavior*, 43, 45–55.

van IJzendoorn, M. H., Feldbrugge, J. T., Derks, F. C., (1997). Attachment representations of personality-disordered criminal offenders. *American Journal of Orthopsychiatry*, 67(3), 449–459.

Verona, E., & Fox, B. (2025). Pathways to crime and antisocial behavior: A critical analysis of psychological research and a call for broader ecological perspectives. *Annual Review of Clinical Psychology*, 21(1), 439–464.

Verona, E., & Vitale, J. (2006). Psychopathy and violence. In C. J. Patrick (Ed.), *Handbook of psychopathy* (pp. 415–432). Guilford Press.

Viding, E., & Larsson, H. (2010). Genetics of child and adolescent psychopathy. In R. T. Salekin & D. R. Lynam (Eds.), *Handbook of child and adolescent psychopathy* (pp. 113–134). Guilford Press.

Volkan, V. D. (1988). *The need to have enemies and allies: From clinical practice to international relationships*. Jason Aronson.

Weeks, R., & Widom, C. S. (1998). Self-report of early childhood victimization among incarcerated adult male felons. *Journal of Interpersonal Violence*, 13(3), 346–361.

Welldon, E. (1988). *Mother, Madonna, whore: The idealization and denigration of motherhood*. Other Press.

Welldon, E. (1996). Group-analytic psychotherapy in an outpatient setting. In C. Cordess & M. Cox (Eds.), *Forensic psychotherapy: Crime, psychodynamics and the offender patient* (pp. 63–82). Jessica Kingsley.

Winnicott, D. W. (1946). Some psychological aspects of juvenile delinquency. In L. Caldwell & H. T. Robinson (Eds.), *The collected works of D. W. Winnicott, vol. 3: 1946–1951* (pp. 43–48). Oxford University Press.

Winnicott, D. W. (1953). Transitional objects and transitional phenomena; a study of the first not-me possession. *International Journal of Psychoanalysis*, 34(2), 89–97.

Winnicott, D. W. (1960). Ego distortion in terms of true and false self. In D. W. Winnicott (Ed.), *The maturational processes and the facilitating environment: Studies in the theory of emotional development* (pp. 140–152). Karnac Books.

Winnicott, D. W. (2016a [1955–1959]). The antisocial tendency. In L. Caldwell & H. T. Robinson (Eds.), *The collected works of D. W. Winnicott: Volume 5, 1955 1959* (pp. 149–158). Oxford Academic.

Winnicott, D. W. (2016b [1968]). Delinquency as a sign of hope. In L. Caldwell & H. T. Robinson (Eds.), *The collected works of D. W. Winnicott: Volume 8, 1967–1968* (pp. 91–98). Oxford Academic.

Wong, S. C., Gordon, A., & Gu, D. (2007). Assessment and treatment of violence-prone forensic clients: An integrated approach. *The British Journal of Psychiatry. Supplement*, 49, s66–s74.

Woodworth, M., Freimuth, T., Hutton, E. L., Carpenter, T., Agar, A. D., & Logan, M. (2013). High-risk sexual offenders: An examination of sexual fantasy, sexual paraphilia, psychopathy, and offence characteristics. *International Journal of Law and Psychiatry*, 36(2), 144–156.

Woodworth, M., & Porter, S. (2002). In cold blood: Characteristics of criminal homicides as a function of psychopathy. *Journal of Abnormal Psychology*, 111(3), 436–445.

Yakeley, J. (2010). *Working with violence – A contemporary psychoanalytic approach*. Palgrave Macmillan.

Yakeley, J. (2022). Treatment for perpetrators of intimate partner violence: What is the evidence? *Journal of Clinical Psychology*, 78(1), 5–14.

Yakeley, J., & Meloy, R. (2012). Understanding violence: Does psychoanalytic thinking matter? *Aggression and Violent Behavior*, 17(3), 229–239.

Yakeley, J., Rost, F., Wood, H., & Abid, S. (2025). Paraphilias, problematic sexual behaviours and personality disorder—To what extent are they linked? *Personality and Mental Health*, 19(1), e1650.

Yang, Y., & Raine, A. (2018). The neuroanatomical bases of psychopathy: A review of brain imaging findings. In C. J. Patrick (Ed.), *Handbook of psychopathy* (2nd edn., pp. 380–400). Guilford Press.
Young, J. E., Klosko, J. S., & Weishaar, M. E. (2003). *Schema therapy: A practitioner's guide.* Guilford Press.

Index

For Product Safety Concerns and Information please contact our EU
representative GPSR@taylorandfrancis.com
Taylor & Francis Verlag GmbH, Kaufingerstraße 24, 80331 München, Germany